*The*
EVERYDAY AYURVEDA
GUIDE TO SELF-CARE

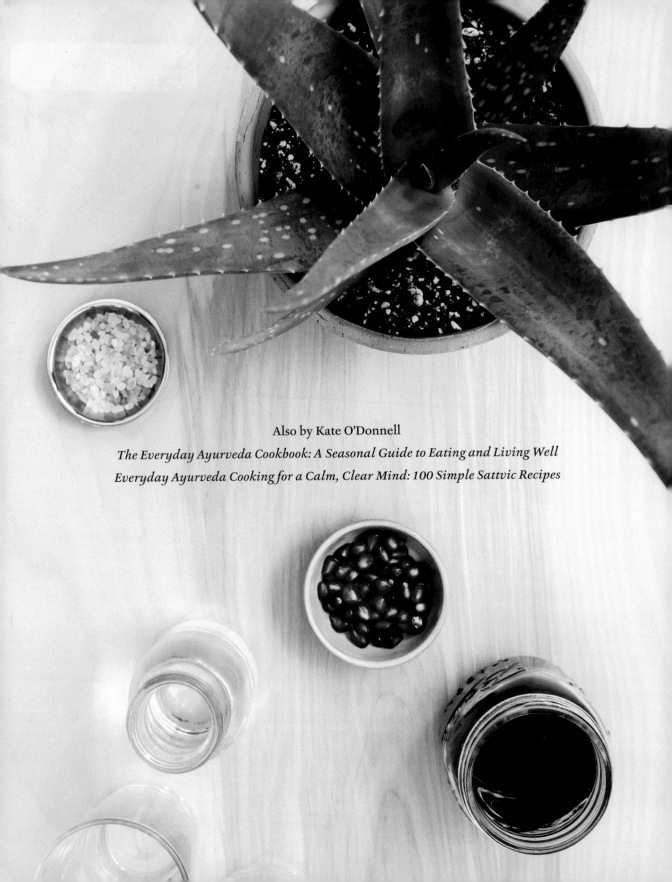

Also by Kate O'Donnell

*The Everyday Ayurveda Cookbook: A Seasonal Guide to Eating and Living Well*

*Everyday Ayurveda Cooking for a Calm, Clear Mind: 100 Simple Sattvic Recipes*

*The*
# EVERYDAY AYURVEDA
# GUIDE TO SELF-CARE

Rhythms, Routines, and Home Remedies for Natural Healing

## KATE O'DONNELL

*Photographs by* CARA BROSTROM

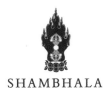

SHAMBHALA

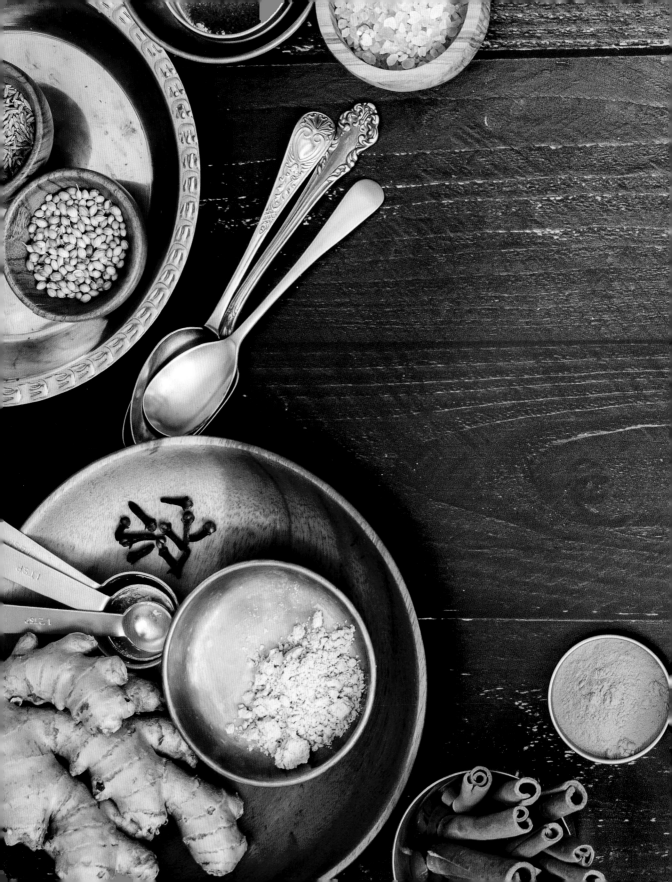

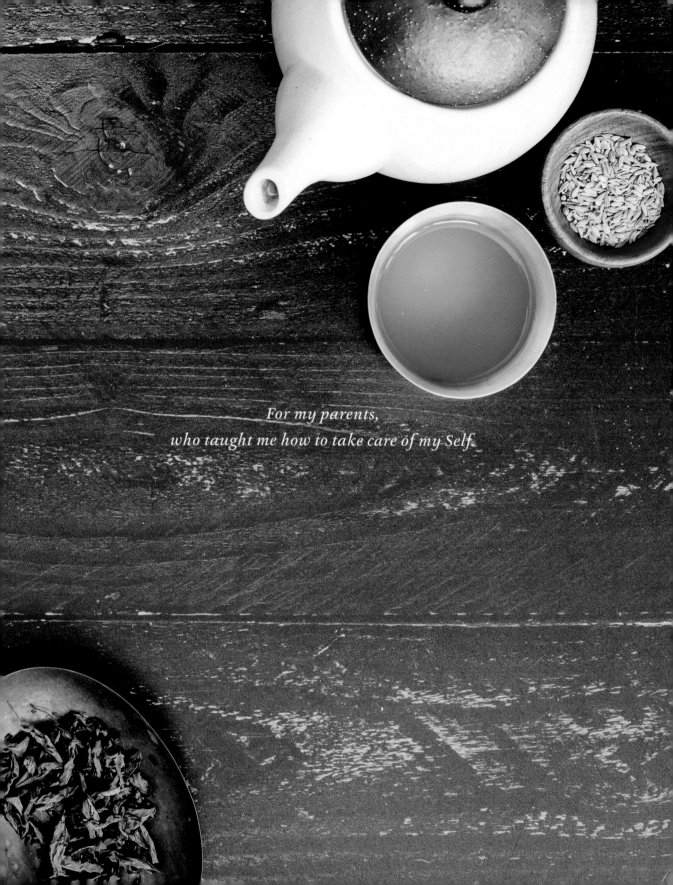

*For my parents,*
*who taught me how to take care of my Self.*

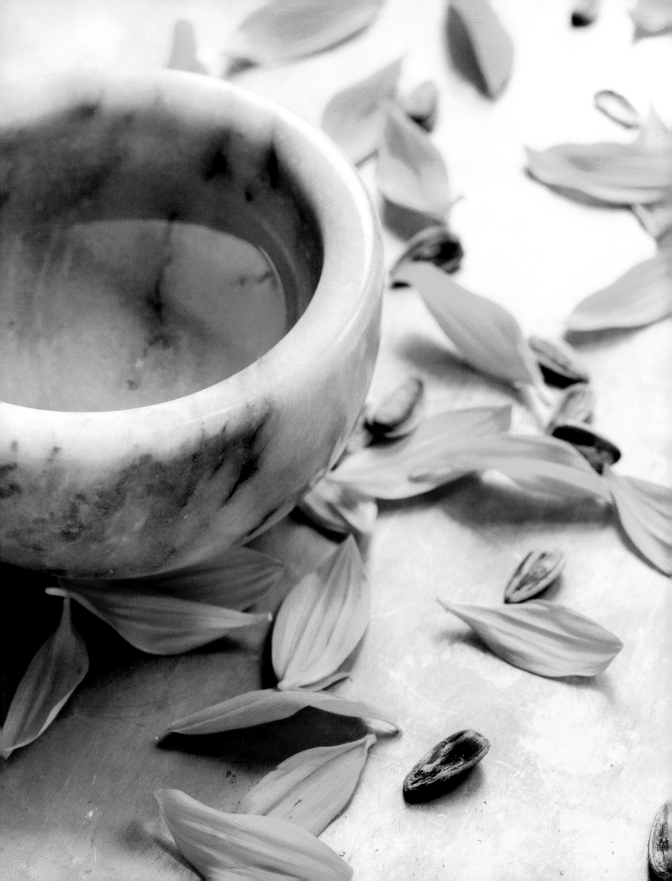

# CONTENTS

# AUTHOR'S NOTE

More than twenty years ago, I journeyed to India on a quest for self-knowledge. I wandered the subcontinent with a backpack, delving into Indian culture, Vedic philosophy, and yoga practice. It was my struggle with parasites that brought me to Ayurveda. The diet and lifestyle practices I learned from doctors in India became my path of self-reliant healing. In this guide to self-care, I offer a process, based on my own experiments with Ayurvedic living, for befriending your body and discovering how best to care for it. It's a unique journey to discover what works for *you*. The launchpad is an ancient body of wisdom, the fruits of collected observations from thousands of years of human trial and error. Join me, dear reader, for a journey into self and into care. It's totally worth your time.

This book offers a new way to think about your health and understand the cause-and-effect relationship between your body, your environment, and your lifestyle. Taking care of yourself is about maintaining good health through a steady practice of self-observation. Ayurveda works when you pay attention to your Self. The information you gain about what makes you glow is pure gold. Think about caring for plants and pets. You have to pay attention to them—figure out what kind of food they like, how much sun and water they need—and watch how they react to changes. Everybody knows you have to walk a dog and water a plant, but how often? Does it change as they age or at different times of year as the amount of sunshine and occurrence of rain shift? There's no judgment if a plant likes less sun or needs fresh soil. And there's no need to judge what makes you thrive, such as needing more rest than exercise or the other way around. There's true intimacy, acceptance, and joy in this kind of self-discovery.

What is special about Ayurveda is the recognition of the central relationship between us and our environment. Human beings are microcosmic members of the macrocosm, and the laws that govern nature govern us as well. For example, waking with the sun and sleeping in the dark have beneficial effects on our health. Modern science is presently fleshing out the details of this phenomenon through the study of circadian rhythms and the effects these rhythms have on our mental well-being, hormones, digestion, and so on.

Ayurveda also takes into account our human nature and the role our minds, emotions, and energies play in our health. There is a subtle reality inside of us that can't be seen or measured but certainly has its effects. Ayurvedic science teaches the art of daily living, of being an integrated, whole person among the needs of job, family, home, and the spiritual heart. It's absolutely possible for anyone to cultivate higher states of health and happiness through the Ayurvedic lifestyle. I've been observing the healing potential of this traditional medicine in all sorts of people, in all sorts of ways, for twenty years. Let's see what it can do for you.

*Your Friend,*
*Kate O'Donnell*

# INTRODUCTION

*The Ayurvedic Definition of Health*

S*wastha* literally means "to be seated in the self" and is loosely defined as "health." This word not only gives us clues about how the system of Ayurveda works to support a long and happy life but also defines the true essence of health. Being seated in the self is like being comfortable in your own skin. To feel at ease in a body requires both physical health and a philosophical sense of OK-ness. Being OK with who we are, with the body we've been given, and with the process of becoming is to be seated in the self. With imbalances like a sour stomach or a disturbed mind, it is more difficult to feel at home in the moment. It's easier to "be here now" when you feel clear. The ancient sages who began the path of Ayurveda pointed out certain aspects of life that are important in the maintenance of swastha.

Ayurveda is defined as the "science of life," but what is life? The root word *ayuh* does not mean simply "life"; it actually describes four aspects that, when combined, form what we call life: the body, the senses, the mind, and the soul.[1] Maintaining good health requires paying equal attention to each of these aspects and respecting their interdependence. Physical wellness, mental wellness, and spiritual wellness are intertwined in this paradigm. To ignore any aspect of life would be to diminish the whole.

The Ayurvedic definition of health goes further to describe the components of health. To be considered a healthy person, each of the following needs to be in balance:

- The functional compounds in the body responsible for movement, transformation, and cohesion (*doshas*)
- Digestive fire (*agni*)
- The seven bodily tissues (*dhatus*)
- The production and elimination of waste (*malas*)
- The sensory and motor organs (*indriyas*)
- The mind (*manas*)
- The soul (*atman*)

In *The Everyday Ayurveda Guide to Self-Care*, we look at taking care of each of these parts of the self. Part one examines the building blocks of the body—the five elements and the three doshas—and how these make up your unique constitution. Part two describes daily and seasonal routines for the preservation of health. Here you learn how to take into account your climate, constitution, and stage of life to create daily and seasonal rhythms that will support you in being your best self. Part three discusses the medicinal qualities of foods, spices, and herbs and how to expand your self-care rituals with home remedies for cleansing, rejuvenation, management of common imbalances, and support of the mind and nervous system.

From the philosophy to the practice, you will learn about the Ayurvedic view of the body and self, as well as how to care for your body, mind, senses, and soul. I know you will feel confident and inspired to begin some self-care routines after understanding the bigger picture of how Ayurveda achieves swastha. Give it some time to gain a slow and steady sense of what your body needs, in real time, and how to deliver the goods. Consider this effort a journey into yourself, which will yield experiential knowledge and the kind of understanding that supports self-healing.

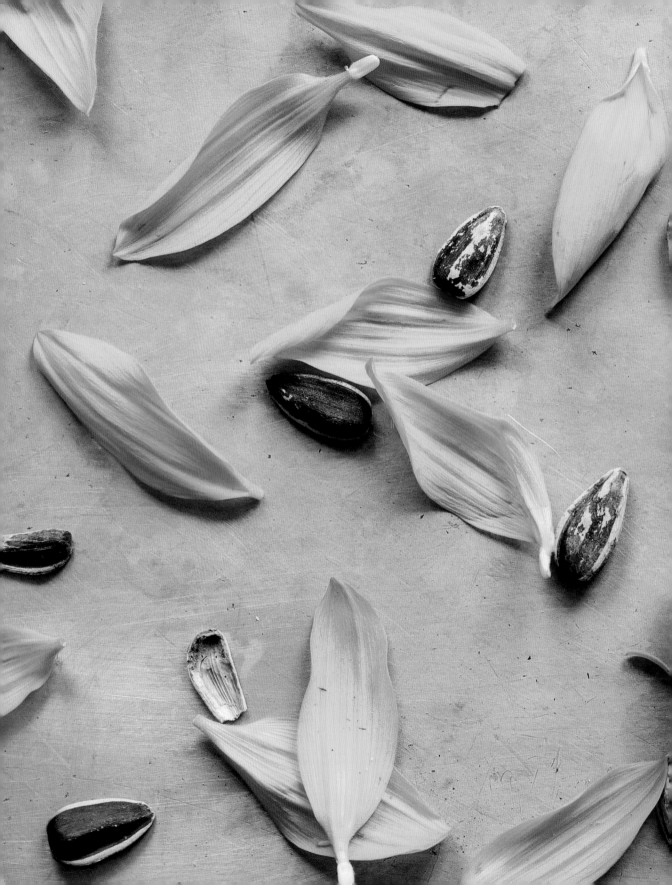

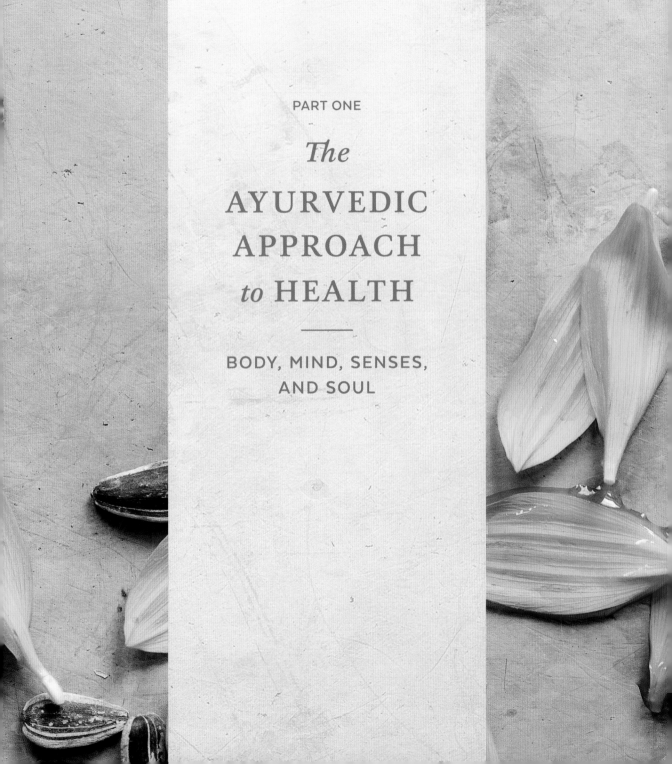

PART ONE

*The*

# AYURVEDIC
# APPROACH
*to* HEALTH

———

BODY, MIND, SENSES,
AND SOUL

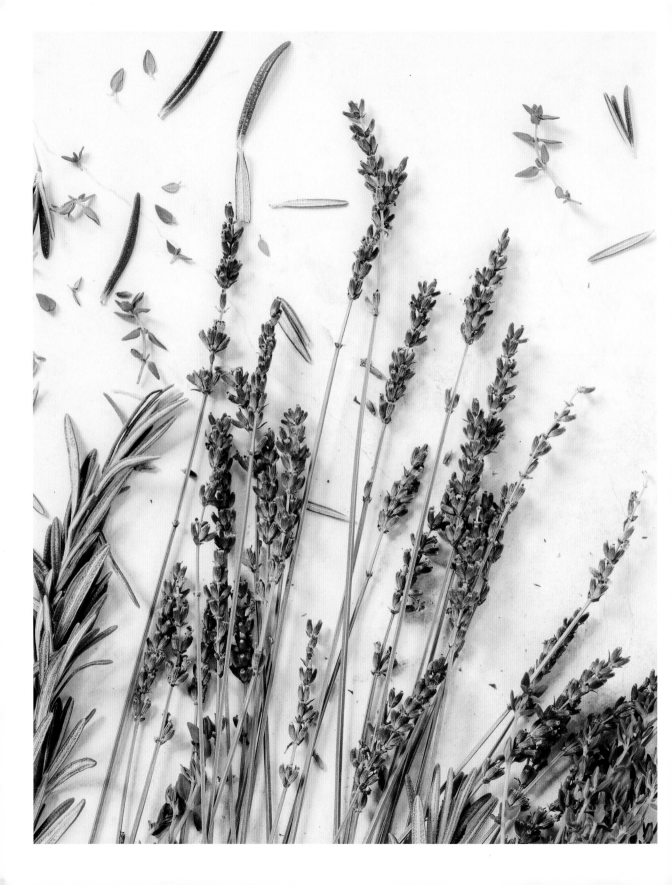

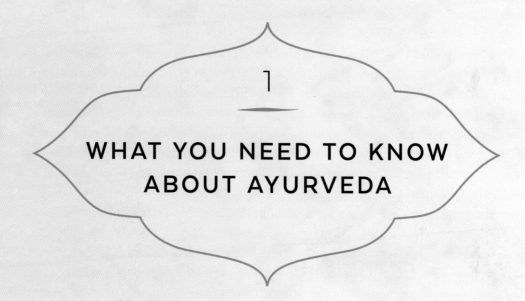

# 1

## WHAT YOU NEED TO KNOW ABOUT AYURVEDA

Welcome to self-care, the Vedic way. This information about health and wellness has philosophical underpinnings that are said to be divinely inspired. Vedic wisdom comes from *rishis*, sages living thousands of years ago who devoted themselves to meditating on the nature of self and universe. The study of this ancient knowledge requires an open mind, as it is your own experience that will reveal the nature of what is true about your unique body/mind/spirit complex. An understanding of Ayurvedic principles encompasses universal truths, which have been discovered by collective human experience over millennia. This way of seeing inevitably expands the mind of the student to hold a truly holistic sense of reality.

The Vedas, India's body of traditional knowledge, cultivated over at least four thousand years, contains not only medical knowledge but also topics such as religious ritual and mantra, music and dance, and architecture. The principal Ayurveda texts—the Charaka Samhita, Sushruta Samhita, and Ashtanga Hrdayam—represent the codification of knowledge gained through ages of human experience that predates the texts. Ayurveda continues to expand and evolve through observation and practice. More recent bodies of work expound further on medical knowledge, but it is compelling how effective the classical information continues to be today. It would seem there are aspects of being human that just don't change, and truths about the nature of Nature that remain true to this day.

The systems of both Ayurveda and yoga emerged from one of the Shad Darshan, the six philosophical views of ancient India. These logical views on the nature of knowledge itself, of the universe, and of humanity's place in it ultimately seek to define a pathway beyond human suffering. If you are reading this book about self-care, it is likely some suffering, or an intelligent wish to avoid future suffering, prompted you to consider looking after your health. It's OK, everybody suffers, according to the sages, so let's not pretend otherwise. Self-care is not all about flower petals and herbal spritzes (though there are some floral recipes in part three). The path to wellness is paved with bricks of self-knowledge, hard-won and wisely applied to the process of daily life.

The Sankhya (pronounced "SAHN-khya"), meaning "number," is the philosophy that informs the paradigms of Ayurveda and yoga. This philosophy names and numbers the constituents of the universe we find ourselves in. It is this makeup of the universe that evolved into the Ayurvedic anatomy of the human system and the laws of action and reaction that govern our passage through this life. Let's take a look, in a practical "how does this affect my life" kind of way. (Hint: keeping an eye on action and reaction is the trick.)

# THE AYURVEDIC FLOW OF LIFE

Ayurveda describes the beginning of life as the interaction of consciousness and matter. This dance gives way to the existence of a universal mind, self-aware individuals, the energies that affect this plane, and its physical building blocks. What gets really interesting is how human beings interact with the world through the organs of perception and the organs of action. Ayurveda and yoga are unique in how they emphasize the importance of these organs, because it is through these gates that energies leave the body, gather information, and set wheels in motion. By observing the activity of these gates, we have some degree of agency over our suffering and our bliss.

### Purusha and Prakriti

*Purusha*, meaning consciousness, is a cosmic concept that transcends space and time. It asserts that consciousness is not limited by matter, but without matter, it is formless. And the world of matter and energy, or *prakriti*, is not sentient without consciousness. The interaction of the two creates sentient beings. Suffering is created when purusha identifies with the limited physical body rather than its own limitless potential. Liberation, the end of a human's suffering state, is to know oneself as limitless and infinite spiritual energy rather than only the body and its trappings. A great example of such liberation is the person with a disease diagnosis who supports the healing process through positive thinking, envisioning and identifying with a reality beyond the disease of the body. Another example is to approach a difficult yoga posture by visualizing a sense of infinite possibility rather than "no way can my body do that." It may still take some practice, but success is far more likely.

Easier said than done. *Maya*—the beguiling world of physicality, its sensory stimulation, and seeds of desire—casts a spell over the purusha. At the heart of Ayurvedic philosophy is a healthy relationship with sensory pleasure and the necessary actions required to undergo a human life without forgetting to connect with the limitless source of vitality: purusha. Unlike yoga, which in some cases renounces sensory pleasure and karma, Ayurveda is for those who wish to maintain good health and vigor to see to the duties and pleasures of life. Many of the practices in this book are designed to maintain physical, as well as spiritual, health in daily life. Like purusha and prakriti, the two are not separate.

## MAHAT, BUDDHI, AND AHAMKARA

Consciousness begins to move in specific ways as matter provides a field in which it can experience itself. This field of universal mind is *mahat*. *Buddhi* is the discriminating mind in human beings. This part of the mind is able to organize and understand information based on experiences and make wise choices. *Ahamkara* is the ego, the part of the mind that identifies as "I" and synthesizes all the information that informs the individual sense of self. It is from this center that we initially act and think. With practice, humans can take a step back and move from buddhi's discernment more often.

## SATTVA, RAJAS, AND TAMAS

*Sattva*, *rajas*, and *tamas* are the energies in the universe that color the mind. Sattva is clear and stable. Rajas is mobile and instigates change and action. Tamas is slow and dull; this energy resists change and is the most earthbound. These three energies are responsible for all movement in the cosmos. Balancing these energies in the mind is necessary to maintain mental clarity and a clear view of reality.

## JNANENDRIYAS

The five senses allow human beings to experience nature and gather information about the external world. They are made of physical as well as subtle attributes. The organs that sense (*jnanendriyas*)—the ears, skin, eyes, tongue, and nose—require subtle energy in order to hear, feel, see, taste, and smell. The mind is, in some schools, considered the sixth sense organ, an organ of cognition that drives as well as digests the activity of the indriyas (senses and motor functions).

Misuse of the senses is a principal factor in the disease process. Generally, overstimulation from excess sensory stimulus adversely affects the mental field and nervous system. Care of the senses is an important part of a daily regimen (described in part two). Cultivating an awareness of these organs and their activity is the first step in moderating their effects on our health.

## KARMENDRIYAS

We use these five parts of the body (*karmendriyas*) to take certain actions that manifest experiences and allow for self-expression.

The mouth is used for speech.
The hands are used for grasping.
The legs and feet are used for walking.
The reproductive organs are used for procreation.
The anus is used for elimination.

Think about the ways we communicate, satisfy desires, move toward and away from things that we like and dislike, make babies, and eliminate waste. These are all hugely important actions, the ramifications of which can change the course of a life. Cultivating an awareness of these actions can help us slow down to consider the big picture and live consciously, rather than acting on impulse and reaping the consequences.

## MAHABHUTAS

The five elements (*mahabhutas*) represent matter in increasing states of density. The subtlest manifestation of prakriti is space. With movement comes air, which has more mass, then heat and then water. The densest element is earth. As density increases, each element becomes more stable, less subtle. For example, we can't see or touch space, but we can see, touch, and smell earth. Different combinations of these elements make up the variations of form in the universe and are the substratum for the Ayurvedic anatomy of the body—the doshas, tissues, and channel system. Ayurveda also categorizes the medicinal properties of substances by their elemental composition and the resulting qualities.

## TANMATRAS

Each of the elements that make up the universe has an essence (*tanmatras*), or root, that can be sensed by human sense organs. These root energies hold the potential for manifestation. For example, sound holds the potential for sensory perception of hearing. If a tree falls in the forest and no one hears it, does it make a sound? Sound requires the ear that hears and the space element in which it vibrates. Air element holds the essence of touch, the movement required to create sensation; fire holds form and light for the eye to see; water holds taste (think saliva); and earth holds smell (think particulate exuding from the earth). The experience of the senses is the key to understanding the elements. Each element, due to its qualities, will manifest as recognizable experiences in the five senses.

The figure on page 8 shows the flow of the Sankhya philosophy. We can see that the body is just one aspect of a larger, interdependent system and that understanding the body has philosophical implications. Being a healthy, happy human requires a strong union of consciousness and matter; a balance of mental energies; and awareness of sensory activity, our actions, and reactions. Whoa! Taking vitamins just won't cut it. This is why the Ayurvedic approach to self-care is so helpful—it addresses all of the components that make up life as we know it.

# SANKHYA PHILOSOPHY

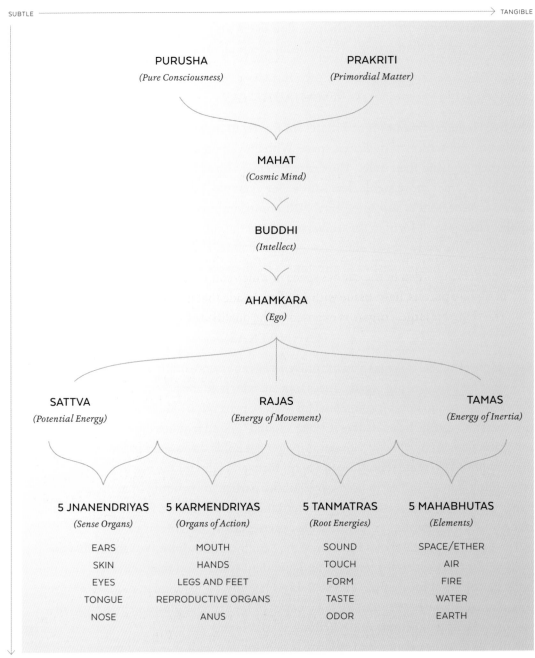

SUBTLE ———————————————————————————→ TANGIBLE

**PURUSHA**
*(Pure Consciousness)*

**PRAKRITI**
*(Primordial Matter)*

**MAHAT**
*(Cosmic Mind)*

**BUDDHI**
*(Intellect)*

**AHAMKARA**
*(Ego)*

**SATTVA**
*(Potential Energy)*

**RAJAS**
*(Energy of Movement)*

**TAMAS**
*(Energy of Inertia)*

| 5 JNANENDRIYAS | 5 KARMENDRIYAS | 5 TANMATRAS | 5 MAHABHUTAS |
| --- | --- | --- | --- |
| *(Sense Organs)* | *(Organs of Action)* | *(Root Energies)* | *(Elements)* |
| EARS | MOUTH | SOUND | SPACE/ETHER |
| SKIN | HANDS | TOUCH | AIR |
| EYES | LEGS AND FEET | FORM | FIRE |
| TONGUE | REPRODUCTIVE ORGANS | TASTE | WATER |
| NOSE | ANUS | ODOR | EARTH |

TANGIBLE

## THE FIVE ELEMENTS AND THE BODY

As we've seen, Ayurveda views the human body, as well as all forms in our universe, as made up of differing combinations of the five elements: space (ether), air, fire, water, and earth.

For example, a body contains space, gases (burps and farts), the heat of fire, the liquidity of water, and its structure—all the tissues and organs—made of earth. A red beet is the same. The sun, the rain, the soil all went into the formation of the beet, and now it is a manifest combination of those elements. Use your body as a frame of reference for understanding the five elements.

### Space

Every body has lots of space in it—usually filled with something like food, acid, fluid, or waste products.

- The large intestine, and indeed the entire digestive channel from the mouth to the anus, is a long, cavernous space. Without that space, where would we put food?
- The delicate organ of the ear has space in which sounds can bounce around.
- Bones are porous, hard tissue with a hollow inside that is filled with marrow.
- The skin, our largest organ, is exposed to the qualities of space all the time.

### Air

Anywhere there is space, there will be air. Space is passive, while air moves around. Anywhere there is movement, there is air. You can feel a breeze on your skin and see it moving the clouds across the sky.

- Respiration is the movement of air in and out of the nose or mouth and into the lungs.
- Passing gas and belching are movements of air out of the intestine and stomach, respectively. If you eat excitedly, more air is likely to get in your mouth, and you will be gassier. Bubbly drinks make you burp because you are ingesting air with your liquid.
- Cracking joints is the sound of air moving out from the spaces between the bones.

### Fire

On earth, anywhere there is heat, there is fire: a hot spring, a lightning bolt, a forest fire. The fire of the sun warms the earth, as it does a human body. The core of the earth is fire, as is the human core—the stomach and small intestine. Anywhere there is heat in the body, it comes from fire.

- The stomach and small intestine contain acids and enzymes that are hot.
- The blood is hot and circulates warmth throughout the body.
- The metabolism and some hormones are hot (as during puberty or pregnancy).
- Eye function requires fire. The eyes are the organs through which light is digested, and without the light of the fire element, sight is not possible.

## Water

Water is all over the planet—in rivers, oceans, the cells of plants, and humans. Water, as you know, makes up 80 percent of the body, and we are filled with liquids.

- All of the mucous membranes that cover the digestive tract, the eyes, and the sinuses rely on water.
- Water is the basis of the lymphatic fluid flowing through your body.
- The blood in your veins contains water.
- Digestive juices require water.
- The synovial fluid that lubricates the joints is part of the water element.
- Saliva is water flowing into the mouth for the first stage of digestion.

## Earth

In nature, earth corresponds to anything solid: soil, rocks, trees, and the flesh of animals. This is the solid structure of the body (all the meaty stuff).

- Adipose tissue (also known as fat) is extra earth element that is stored in the body.
- Muscle fiber is the earth element that holds the skeleton in place.
- The stable part of the bones (not the space inside) that constitutes the structure of the skeleton is made of earth element.
- Organs are made of the earth element.

It's important to remember that the same five elements move around in all of us and in all of nature. We are all made of the same stuff, and Ayurveda views the human organism as a microcosm of the whole universe. When you ingest a rejuvenating tonic at the right time, when you have strong digestion to transform it, when you absorb and assimilate its elements into your tissues, then your body takes the nourishing aspects of water, earth, and other elements from the tonic's ingredients and incorporates them into your structure. The journey of elements from the creation of rejuvenating ingredients to the creation of human tissues unites your body with the ongoing activity of the universe. Circle of life!

## THE THREE DOSHAS

Most people who have heard of Ayurveda have heard of the doshas. These are the functional compounds that arise naturally when the five elements come together, into three pairs, to make up a human organism. *Dosha* literally means "that which is at fault." [1] But doshas aren't a problem until an imbalance has been hanging around for a while. In their normal states, these energies maintain health in the body, but they damage the body if they are in abnormal states. That's why it is more important to understand how to maintain balance than it is to dwell on the doshas as the bad guys.

The three doshas are known as *vata* (that which moves), *pitta* (that which transforms), and *kapha* (that which brings cohesion). Each performs a specific function in the body and manifests as a recognizable grouping of qualities in the body, mind, and emotions. They exist all over the body, but due to the prevalence of elements in certain places, each of the doshas has sites where it is more common and governs local functions. Generally early signs in these sites or functions alert us to an abnormality, such as an increase in gas, anxiety or irritability, acid indigestion, congestion, or a heavy feeling in the stomach. If a body has more of certain elements by nature, some of these symptoms will be more familiar than others. If the trajectory of a dosha does not shift, the abnormality can eventually begin to cause damage to the body.

The doshas can become abnormal in three ways:

1. Quality, as when the moist quality of kapha increases, causing congestion
2. Quantity, as when the air element of vata increases in the colon, causing gas and bloating
3. Function, as when the mental function of pitta to focus the mind goes into overdrive, leading to obsessive thoughts

The doshas are essentially groups of qualities that, due to their nature, hang out together and lend themselves to specific bodily functions. For example, if it's cold out, the skin will eventually become dry. If it's moist out, the skin will become soft. Vata dosha is both dry and cold. Kapha is both moist and soft. Always be sure when you are picturing a dosha, and how it is in a body, to imagine its qualities.

# THE LAW OF OPPOSITES

Our world is made up of coexisting opposites. Like increases like, and opposites balance each other. The twenty qualities, or *gunas*, are how nature keeps a balance, and recognizing and working with the qualities means you can help nature stay on course.

The gunas are the different attributes inherent in all substances. A rock is hard, and a cloud is soft—it's common sense, if you think about it. Pairs of opposing attributes define the way we feel and understand our world through comparison: something's hot or it's cold; it's sharp or it's smooth. Ayurveda has identified ten pairs of opposites that are most useful in medicine. When a quality, or group of qualities, is in excess (it can also be depleted, but excess is more likely), imbalance can occur.

A pile of hot, sharp wasabi paste without any cooling, smooth rice intuitively sounds a little off, doesn't it? Ayurveda encourages balance by introducing qualities opposite to those causing the imbalance, while reducing similar qualities. For instance, in winter you might enjoy a bit of spicy food to warm you up, but you avoid it in summer when the weather is already hot. All of the substances used as medicine (plants, meats, fruits, minerals) as well as our activities have an effect on the body, which is experienced as one or more of the qualities. Picture it: spicy food makes you feel hot and sweaty—the effect of spicy food is heating and oily. Limeade cools and refreshes you—the effect of lime is cool and light.

Once you start to think of your body's sensations or imbalances in terms of the qualities you are experiencing, you will be able to apply remedies by introducing substances that have a balancing effect, whether it's food, spices, or the concentrated qualities of herbs.

The qualities are divided into two opposing categories: building (*brmhana*) and reducing (*langhana*). The balance between these two energies in the body is central to maintaining an even keel, balanced doshas and tissues, and smooth-moving bodily processes.

Building qualities are anabolic. They build mass and nourish the tissues, encourage moisture, and strengthen, ground, and stabilize the body, mind, and nerves. They are found in substances that make the body feel warm, cozy, and safe. The rejuvenating tonic remedies in chapter 10 are excellent examples. They contain milk, nuts and seeds, dates, unctuous herbs, and natural sweeteners. The herbal ghee recipes also contain brmhana qualities.

Reducing qualities are catabolic. They reduce mass and the tissues, eliminate excess water and mucus, and put a spring in your step. Light substances feel refreshing, invigorating, and energizing. Herbal waters are a great example, especially with warming spices such as *ajwain* and tulsi. The *kashayam* remedy section contains several light formulas that use lemon, ginger, clove, and other hot and drying spices. Many of the medicinal food recipes also have light qualities, with cleansers such as dandelion soup, *kanjee*, and *rasam*.

# THE TEN QUALITIES AND THEIR OPPOSITES

In translating Sanskrit, it sometimes takes more than one English word to describe the felt quality. This is why some of the qualities list more than one word. You will also notice that several of the qualities result as much from *activities* (in italics) as from ingesting substances.

| | |
|---|---|
| **Heavy:** Heavy substances can feel like bricks or like good medicine, depending on the preparation and the condition of the digestion when the substance comes down the tube. Heavy substances digest best when they are taken warm, with a bit of spice (imagine the effect of cold fondue). Examples are *shatavari, ashwagandha*, milk, ghee, and dates. *Most sedentary activities produce a heavy quality.* | **Light:** Light substances are generally clarifying and easy to digest, such as broth, herbal teas, watery vegetables, *brahmi*, *triphala*, and *pippali*. A light quality is encouraged by invigorating movement, such as dance parties, and *vigorous exercise.* |
| **Slow/dull:** Heavy substances that digest slowly or activities that make the body and mind feel dull make up this category. Examples include fried foods, beef, drugs, *overeating*, and *oversleeping.* | **Sharp/penetrating/quick:** Think about things that clear your sinuses in a hurry, make your appetite sharp, or help you think straight. Examples are bay leaf, ginger, pickles, rosemary, and cayenne, as well as activities that keep the mind and reflexes sharp, such as *nasal irrigation (neti)*, Sudoku, and *sports.* |
| **Cool:** A cool quality is introduced by things that not only are cool when you ingest them but have a cooling aftereffect. When you eat or drink cooling substances, you are likely to feel cold or refreshed. Examples are the aloe cooler recipes, brahmi, dandelion, cilantro, mint, cucumber, and coconut. Activities include *swimming* and *relaxing.* | **Hot:** Substances with a heating aftereffect, such as lemon, pepper, cayenne, honey, and garlic, are featured in cough and cold remedies. Anything that causes acid indigestion will be heating, including coffee and tomatoes. Activities that get you all worked up can also be heating, like *feisty competition, hot yoga*, and *stressing out.* |
| **Oily/unctuous:** Humid weather can make you feel oily—think moisture. All substances containing natural oils, such as coconut, nuts, fish, seeds, milk, and olives, can promote this quality. Moist herbs such as ashwagandha, shatavari, and licorice are unctuous. Activities that increase moisture are *swimming, sitting in a steam room*, and *oil massage.* | **Dry:** Some substances, such as tea, coriander, and turmeric, absorb water from the body and contain no or little oil, giving them a drying effect. Other examples include beans, caffeine, and barley. Activities that are dry and reduce moisture include *dry brushing, saunas*, and *time spent at a high altitude.* |

| | |
|---|---|
| **Smooth:** Smooth substances are soft and moist. Ingesting substances with this quality will smooth the skin as well as the intestines. Examples include eggplant, chia, licorice, avocado, and banana. *Oil massage* and *swimming* are two activities with this quality. | **Rough:** Rough substances require lots of chewing and digestive fire. Examples are corn chips, coarse flours, and celery sticks and other raw vegetables. Activities that promote this quality include *jogging in the cold* and *very vigorous exercise.* |
| **Dense/solid:** Dense substances contain fats and moisture such as eggplant, ghee, and yogurt. Stable activities include *sitting around* and *watching TV.* | **Liquid:** Density is diluted by a liquid quality. Some substances, such as water, coconut water, and milk, are obviously liquid. A substance can be rendered less dense by watering it down, such as going from cream to skim milk, or yogurt to *takra.* All of the herbal waters and kashayam recipes are liquid. *Exercise* dilutes density in the body by mobilizing the blood. |
| **Soft:** A soft quality makes the body and attitude gentle, supple, and moist. All substances can be softened by cooking them and adding liquid. Unctuous substances are generally soft; examples include licorice, shatavari, and ghee. Activities that calm the body and mind include *oil massage, hugging,* and *gentle yoga.* | **Hard:** A hard quality makes the body strong, stiff, and dry. Hard substances include raw vegetables, dehydrated substances, and gingerroot. Wind and cold weather can increase hard quality, as can activities that build muscle and reduce fat, such as *aerobics* and *body building.* |
| **Stable:** A stable quality feels safe, comfortable, and steady. Substances that increase stable quality will be nourishing to the dhatus, such as rejuvenating tonics and herbal ghees. Salt increases stability by holding water in the body. Activities that establish rhythm, such as *daily morning or evening routines, consistent meal-times,* and *staying in one place,* are stable. | **Mobile/unstable:** This quality is present in substances and activities that increase circulation, such as rosemary, tulsi, turmeric, hot peppers, spicy honey, and *travel* or *relocation.* |
| **Cloudy/slimy:** A cloudy quality is present in substances that are opaque or translucent, such as coconut milk, almond milk, and creamy soups. *Using drugs, prescription or otherwise,* and *alcohol* increases a cloudy quality. | **Clear:** Aloe vera and herbal waters are clear. Substances that are hot and penetrating, such as clove, pepper, and mustard seed, have a clearing quality as well. Some activities such as *meditation* and *deep breathing* clear the mind. |
| **Gross/big:** *Gross* means "of the physical body, the material world." The gross body includes all of our tissues and wastes. Gross quality is especially present in meat. *Focusing the mind on the physical body* only increases the gross quality. | **Subtle/small:** "Subtle quality" can refer to something minute like a cell or molecule, or to the energy body and mind. Brahmi has an affinity for the subtle body and mind. *Spiritual practice* and *prayer* represent subtle activities. |

## The Qualities of Vata

Where there is space, air will move, and the compound qualities of space and air manifest as cold, light, dry, rough, mobile, erratic, and clear. Space and air have no heat, wetness, or heaviness. These qualities are inherent in fire, water, and earth.

The qualities of space and air are naturally going to act a certain way and have certain effects on the body. Think of vata ("VA-tah") as the currents of the body. The body knows that food goes in the mouth, then down and out. Vata ushers it along. There is nothing problematic about the qualities of space and air or their function. However, if a body has accumulated too much of these qualities, certain aspects can get out of balance. For instance, autumn gets windy, dry, and cold, and then so does the body after a little while (unless, of course, you are taking care to keep warm, eat warm moist foods, and drink warm water). Too many vata qualities can result in signs of imbalance such as gas and constipation, increasingly dry skin, racing thoughts, and anxiety.

| Healthy vata ensures that the body has | Too many vata qualities may cause |
| --- | --- |
| Consistent elimination | Gas and constipation |
| Free breathing | Asthma |
| Good circulation | Cold hands and feet |
| Keen senses | Anxiety / feeling overwhelmed |
| Creativity | |

## The Qualities of Pitta

Where there is fire, there has to be water to keep it from burning everything up. The resulting compound is firewater, a liquid, hot, sharp, penetrating, light, mobile, oily, smelly grouping of qualities (think acid or bile). When food gets chewed, pitta ("PITT-ah") moves in to break it down, liquidize it, metabolize it, and transform it into tissues. No problem with that—unless, of course, your insides get too hot or too sharp, which can result in signs of imbalance such as acidy burps or reflux, diarrhea, skin rashes, or inflammation.

| Healthy pitta creates | Too many pitta qualities may cause |
|---|---|
| Good appetite and metabolism | Acid indigestion or reflux |
| Steady hormones | Dysmenorrhea |
| Sharp eyesight | Red, dry eyes and/or the need for glasses |
| Ease of comprehension | Tendency to overwork |
| Good complexion (rosy skin) | Acne, rosacea |
| | Irritability |
| | Competitiveness |

## The Qualities of Kapha

Only when you add water to sand does it stick together so you can build a castle. The earth element requires water in the same way to hold the body together. Kapha ("CUP-hah") is like glue: cool, liquid, slimy, heavy, slow, dull, dense, and stable. This grouping of qualities provides density in the bones and fat, cohesion in the tissues and joints, and plenty of mucus so we don't dry out. Great! Unless the body becomes too heavy and too sticky, which can result in signs of imbalance such as loss of appetite, slow digestion, sinus troubles and allergies, or weight gain.

| Healthy kapha provides | Too many kapha qualities may cause |
|---|---|
| Strong bodily tissues | Weight gain |
| Well-lubricated joints and mucous membranes | Water retention |
| Hearty immune system | Sinus or lung congestion |
| | Lethargy and sadness |

To put all the pieces together, look at the sites and functions of the doshas illustrated in the figure on page 18. Imagine an increase in the qualities or quantity of a dosha, in its sites, and what that might feel like. Think about how these qualities are important for bodily functions to be carried out. Slow down and take a few minutes to really feel for them in your body. Again, some of the qualities will be more familiar than others. This is a clue to understanding your constitution.

For example, you know pitta resides in the midsection of the body and is hot, sharp, and penetrating. Imagine things getting hotter in your stomach and/or small intestine. This might manifest as acid stomach, hot poops, or an overheated, prickly, burning sensation in the midsection. We also know kapha predominates in the upper portion of the body. Imagine an increase in moist, dense, heavy qualities in your mouth, stomach, sinuses, or lungs. This might create a loss of appetite and a heavy feeling in your stomach, sniffles, thick snots, a wet cough, or even the feeling of a heavy heart. Vata predominates in the lower abdomen. Imagine an increase in air's cold, light, dry, hard qualities; the belly might feel cool and hard to the touch and appear bloated.

Having a little information about the doshas, their qualities, their normal functions, and a few basic signs and symptoms of imbalance can help you know what to watch out for, as well as which diet and lifestyle choices are most beneficial for you. The qualities are the things to recognize: look beyond the symptom to the qualities that are causing it. For example, why does constipation often result from air travel? The dry quality of the pressurized cabin increases the dry quality in your body. Knowing this, you can make sure to pack an oil for massage or an herbal ghee to have with hot milk at bedtime and avoid dry foods such as crackers and popcorn. Similarly, healthy mucus lubricates the membranes, but if there's too much of it or it's too sticky, you have problems. Since the qualities of mucus are moist, sticky, and thick, you should go for something like a spice-infused honey rather than ice cream if your sweet tooth strikes.

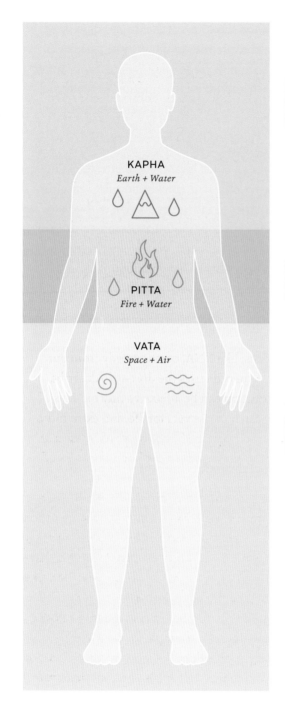

**KAPHA**
*Earth + Water*

**PITTA**
*Fire + Water*

**VATA**
*Space + Air*

## LOCATIONS AND FUNCTIONS OF THE DOSHAS

**KAPHA** is the energy of structure and lubrication together; cohesion (think "glue").
*Earth + Water*

Kapha is most prevalent in the head and chest, as well as the upper stomach and the fatty tissue. It is responsible for maintaining memory and the physical structure and immunity of the body, as well as providing moisture in the stomach and mouth, sinuses, lungs, and joints.

**PITTA** is the energy of transformation.
*Fire + Water*

Pitta is most prevalent around the midsection, specifically the stomach and small intestine, and the blood. It is responsible for digestion and absorption, cognition, eyesight, and maintaining warmth and skin complexion in the body.

**VATA** is the energy of movement.
*Space + Air*

Vata is most prevalent below the navel, specifically in the colon, rectum, bladder, thighs, low back, and legs. It is responsible for elimination, urination, menstruation, and circulation, as well as the activity of the sense organs.

# THE SEVEN CONSTITUTIONAL TYPES

One of my favorite words, *prakriti* literally means "beginning of creation." It is the original nature or essence of something manifest. This can be applied to describe the nature of the physical world, made of the five elements and enlivened by subtle energies. The human body is also like this, made of the five elements and subtle energies. Whether we are talking about the macrocosm or the microcosm, prakriti is the same concept. Every body has a unique original physical makeup. There is no "one size fits all" in Ayurveda, which promotes an understanding and acceptance of the elemental makeup of your body and how to work with this truth for optimal wellness. One person moves quickly, another slowly; one person runs hot, another cold. Neither is better or worse. For everything in this universe, there are strengths and weaknesses. It is common to think one thing is "better" than another, but of course, it depends. If you are hiking Mount Everest, you will have an easier time of it if you are the hot type. If you are in the desert, you are lucky if you are the cold type. Knowing your own strengths and weaknesses helps you support your body and mind through an appropriate lifestyle rather than one imposed on your body without consideration.

The body's constitution, or makeup of elements, like DNA, comes mostly from our parents. Elements compound into doshas, and Ayurveda uses the doshas to describe prakriti. In the first seven years of life, the constitution can be affected a tiny bit. Lots of movement or physical and emotional instability can increase vata for life, and extremities of diet and climate also affect the elements in the body during formative years. After that point, it is fixed. Doshas can go up and down, but the baseline of the body, its intended state of being, has been set.

It is important to know your prakriti because the qualities of that dosha will be more prevalent in your body. For example, a kapha type can expect more heavy, moist qualities, which may cause sensitivity to dairy because it is heavy and moist. This knowledge can inform your choices about diet, exercise, and daily routines. People who are "tridoshic" have an even balance of all three doshas and generally enjoy better health. Those who have one or two primary doshas may experience imbalances of the same dosha(s).

Most bodies have two prevalent doshas, not just one. It may be easier to identify a dosha in the constitution during the season of similar qualities. For example, kapha will show up in rainy weather rather than in a hot, dry summer, which reduces kapha. If your constitution is very dry, rain will be a relief, but if your constitution is mainly kapha, rain will aggravate it and you may feel stuffy, heavy, and slow.

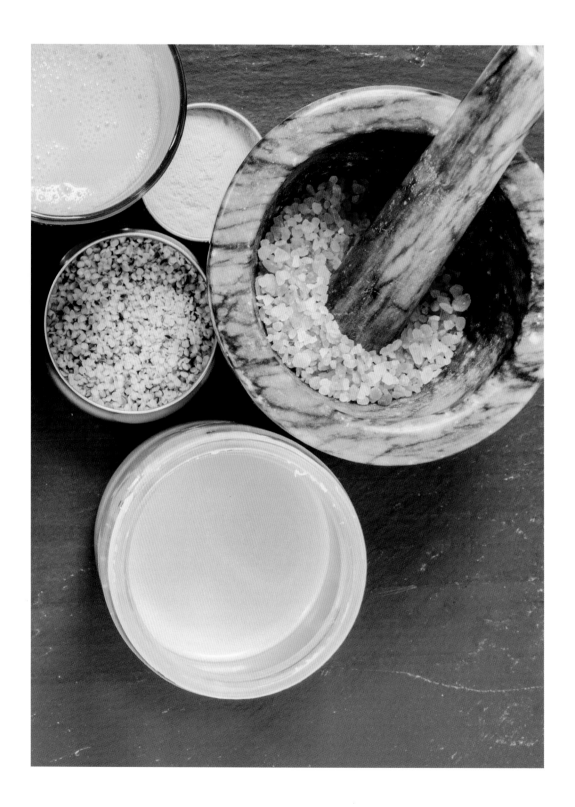

Seasonal changes can make identifying your constitution a little more confusing. Observe how the seasons affect you over at least one annual cycle. See how changes in your seasonal routines may create changes in your body and mind and be open to new ideas about your prakriti. For example, you might feel quite dry in winter and gravitate toward sesame oil massage and toast with lots of ghee. But when the thaw comes and you hit some rainy weather, do you still feel dry? You might notice you don't need sesame oil on your skin anymore to stay supple. Instead, you may feel like dry brushing and making a dandelion soup. Or maybe you notice dryness all year round and that sesame oil always feels appropriate.

The following list describes the seven constitutional types. Pure vata, pitta, or kapha types are far less common than constitutions with two doshas:

- VATA types are cold, dry, and light. They need to oil the body, eat good fats, and get enough rest.
- PITTA types are intense, hot, and sharp. They need to eat calming, cooling foods, make time for R&R, and avoid overdoing both work and play.
- KAPHA types are slow, moist, and stable. They may to need to shake it up a bit from time to time with spontaneity or travel, eat lighter foods, and be sure to exercise.
- VATA-PITTA types often need to keep the air element pacified, because if it blows erratically on the fire, it may cause unstable, dry, and hot qualities in the body as well as in the emotions. This is a subtle combination with an affinity for the mind. The drive of pitta can overwhelm the sensitivity of vata. Generally, staying grounded and well rested is the key.
- PITTA-KAPHA types are very strong, but there can be a lot of water in the constitution. Damp, cloudy weather and too much fatty, oily food can cause imbalances. Sometimes the appetite is stronger than the metabolism, which can result in weight gain, especially around the middle, and clogging of the channels.
- VATA-KAPHA types are lacking in fire and need to eat according to appetite; stick with easy-to-digest, warm, nicely spiced foods, and stay mobile, focused, and motivated.
- TRIDOSHIC Tridoshic types are an even balance of the five elements. They tend to be healthier, have an easier time making wise choices, and do well with basic daily self-care routines and simple seasonal variations.

The table on page 24 summarizes the elements, best and worst seasons, and good self-care habits for each of the doshas and dosha combinations. (The actual self-care routines are described in part two.)

## Identifying Your Prakriti

I often hear people say two things when they are working with prakriti: (1) "I want to know what my dosha is" and (2) "I don't understand the quiz questions; the result is different every time I take it." Many modern Ayurveda reference books and websites contain a "dosha quiz" with questions about your physical, mental, emotional, and behavioral profile. For example, do you have thick or thin hair, do you have a good memory or not so much, are you a sound or light sleeper, and so on. I find that people's answers to these questions are often not relative to the bigger picture. You may think you are a light sleeper because you wake up nightly to pee, but until you meet someone who wakes up when a breeze comes in the window, you don't really know what light sleep is. Maybe you wake up to pee because you forget to drink water all day and then overdo it before bed as a last resort. You're not *really* a light sleeper. The questions, taken out of context, can be confusing or misleading. So, we are not doing the dosha quiz here, folks.

I've given you a good deal of context about each of the doshas, their qualities, how they act, and how they can combine into different constitutional types. Rather than try to peg yourself as a certain "type" and dutifully follow the dos and don'ts for your dosha, I'd like you to practice self-observation. Over time, the activity of the three doshas and the presence of their qualities in your body will reveal themselves. Consider their locations, their qualities, their respective seasons, and the jobs they do in your body. Do some sleuthing. It's not always obvious (although sometimes it actually is). Try any or all of the following suggestions to get going, and give it some time:

- **Keep a journal.** If you aren't the type to remember what you did a few days ago, keeping a simple journal about your experiences can give you a point of reference. For example, you may note, "This spring I felt a little depressed. I also noticed dairy made me feel heavy, and it doesn't always do that." Go back monthly or seasonally and refresh your memory about any health concerns, digestive changes, and seasonal changes to physical or mental health. This can help you identify recurring patterns. Congestion or mood swings, for example, can suggest an imbalanced dosha. If it comes back over and over, you can't just chalk it up to your work or the weather. Notice if the symptom comes back at certain times of year or is triggered by certain foods. Think about the qualities of that food or season; which dosha(s) are those qualities similar to? You may always come up with the same answer, and this is because of your prakriti.

- **Talk to people.** Gain some context by asking other people what *their* sleep or digestion is like, what state of mind (fast or slow) they have, what their least and most preferred kind of weather is. Compare and contrast your own experiences.
- **Observe seasonal changes and their effects.** The more you are affected by the qualities of a season, the more likely it is that these qualities predominate in your own body to begin with. Give yourself a full annual cycle to pay attention to changes.
- **Observe the effects food and drink have on you.** If cold, dry, and mobile don't agree with you—for example, beans make you gassy, iced drinks make you shiver, and you have a hard time sitting still—think vata. If hot, sharp, and irritable have got your number—for example, orange juice and tomato sauce give you acid stomach—think pitta. If you tend toward heavy, moist, and slow—where lack of exercise or dense food equal weight gain—think kapha.
- **Think back in time.** If you have some toxins built up, it can look a lot like kapha. If you have inflammation, it can seem like pitta. Anxiety, no matter the cause, can feel like vata. But in any of these cases, the expected dosha may not be to blame. Try to remember your tendencies from when you were a kid (or ask a family member). Before so many factors took hold, what kind of food did you gravitate toward when given the choice? Did you have any food sensitivities? If it were up to you, did you prefer to be active or sedentary? Did you experience any of the signs and symptoms attributed to one or more of the doshas when you were young? I sometimes watch kids on the playground or at the beach. I observe the different body types and behaviors—things are so clear in little ones. If you have kids, you can see reflections of your body's tendencies repeating in them. Lots of clues!

When in doubt, see a practitioner. If you feel like it's getting complicated, or you have some imbalances that need to be addressed before you can begin to see yourself clearly, getting some help saves time. There are so many interwoven factors in the fabric that makes up your life. The good news is that some of it is predictable. Someone who spends a lot of time observing life's patterns can help you make sense of your own patterns, understand your strengths, and suggest things to watch out for.

## KEY CHARACTERISTICS OF THE SEVEN CONSTITUTIONS

| Prakriti | Elements | Worst Season | Best Season | Key Self-Care Routines |
|---|---|---|---|---|
| VATA | Air + space | Winter | Summer | Oil massage, *nasya* (oiling the nose) |
| PITTA | Fire + water | Summer | Fall | Head massage with coconut oil, contemplation, and relaxation |
| KAPHA | Earth + water | Spring | Summer | Dry brushing, *neti* (nasal irrigation) |
| VATA-PITTA | Space + air + fire + water | Fall | Spring | Oil massage, especially the head and feet |
| PITTA-KAPHA | Fire + water (×2) + earth | Spring | Fall | Exercise |
| VATA-KAPHA | Space + air + water + earth | Winter | Summer | Hot water with lemon, largest meal at midday |
| TRIDOSHIC | Space + air + fire + water + earth | Balanced | Balanced | Balanced seasonal regimens |

It's easy to focus on dosha, that which is at fault. But categorizing yourself as a dosha ("I'm so vata") or identifying yourself with states of imbalance is not the aim of Ayurvedic wisdom. Remember that the doshas are functional friends that maintain health in the body and bring certain qualities and energies to the physical and mental spheres. They are also like "mindfulness bells" that give us signs when we are living out of balance.

### States of Imbalance

Speaking of living out of balance, what about when you suspect you are out of balance already? *Vikruti* is a current state of imbalance, where the doshas are not in their original state but have undergone changes in quality, quantity, or function. This can be a short-term or long-term thing. For example, kapha vikruti can arise on a rainy day and ease when the sun comes out. The effects of five years at a desk job with no exercise and very little sunshine, however, are not going to go away with one sunny day. Think of vikruti as having a half-life. It may take half as long as the imbalance has been around to resolve it, so in the case of that desk job, it will be around two-plus years. It may be less or more because many factors are involved, but this is the general idea.

## VATA PROBLEMS

Vata is the dosha most likely to go out of whack. This is because its nature is to move and change; it is unstable. Sensory stimulus also plays a large part in vata imbalances these days, and those who "live large" or live in urban centers are likely to have some degree of vata vikruti. Many of the self-care practices and routines in part two are intended to balance this problem.

I often hear, "What if I'm not sure what my prakriti is and what's an imbalance?" Well, say, gas and bloating are plaguing you; it makes sense to address that regardless. In a general sense, if a symptom is bothersome, managing it is going to eventually reveal the true nature beneath the imbalance. Like I said, understanding prakriti and vikruti can take some time.

Doshas that have undergone changes need to be addressed by Ayurvedic practitioners and doctors. Prevention is one thing, but if imbalance is long-term or chronic, it's a good idea to consult a professional, which can save you from making things worse.

## IMBALANCE AND DISEASE

*Samprapti* means "progression of imbalance." Even a deeply rooted and symptomatically complicated disease begins with stages of imbalance. Having the awareness and the tools to recognize and address early signs and symptoms of imbalance is the name of the prevention game. Samprapti has six stages:

1. Accumulation of dosha
2. Provocation or aggravation
3. Spread
4. Depositing or localizing in a weak area
5. Manifestation
6. Destruction, structural changes

Knowing how doshas get from accumulation all the way to disease breaks it down a bit and illuminates the importance of listening to early signs and symptoms.

In the first three stages, the quantity of one or more of the doshas and their qualities increases. In the latter three stages, qualitative changes occur, which means the imbalance damages certain tissues of the body. In the first three stages, managing excess doshas will change the course, or progression, of the imbalance, but the later three stages become more difficult to heal due to structural tissue changes. Ayurveda texts describe specific signs for each stage. While Ayurveda does address serious disease states, this goes beyond the scope of our discussion here. In the table on page 27 are examples of low-key symptoms in earlier stages, to illustrate how imbalances progress.

An Ayurvedic doctor may be able to help address imbalances in later stages of development, but in this book, we will focus on recognizing and managing the first three stages. Keep thinking of doshas as groups of elements and qualities. Think about how a group of qualities might manifest the symptoms mentioned. How does heat go from indigestion to acid reflux? How could a loss of appetite lead to nausea? The qualities are sensory, so if you practice paying attention, you can begin to understand early signs through your own experience, knowing what is normal and not normal.

General self-care, healthy diet, and daily and seasonal routines are meant to keep imbalances from progressing beyond the first two stages. Making wise choices keeps us from increasing certain qualities that may be on the rise and are likely prevalent in the constitution to begin with. Balancing the six tastes in the diet, for example, assures we are getting a balance of all the elements. (The six tastes are discussed in detail in chapter 8.) Choosing the right oils to apply to the skin can warm, cool, or stimulate, as needed. The Ayurvedic diet and lifestyle are a synergy of routines and helpful foods, spices, and herbs that keep our elements in balance.

### The Three Causes of Imbalance

Ayurveda recognizes three main causes of disease and imbalance, which are collectively called *trividha karana*. If you manage these three areas well, your body and mind should remain in a state of relative balance, and the progression from imbalance to disease will not occur. The three factors are:

1. **Kala:** Time of day and time of year (seasonal affect)
2. **Karma:** Actions and activities pertaining to body, speech, and mind[2]
3. **Artha samyoga:** Too much or too little use of the sense organs

THE WISDOM OF TIME. *Kala*, time, is an expansive concept, like consciousness, that defies simple explanation. Unlike the human body, time doesn't have a beginning or an end. Time is eternal and continuous, and even the planets are subject to it. Where life is concerned, time is responsible for birth and death and all of the changes that take place in between. Everything in the universe is undergoing a continual process of transformation. In other words, change is the only constant.

## THE SIX STAGES OF DISEASE

| Stage | Description | Symptoms | Example |
|---|---|---|---|
| Accumulation | A dosha begins to increase in its own site, like kapha in the stomach or vata in the colon. Something might feel not quite right, but there aren't any manifestations yet. | Vata: bloating<br>Pitta: slight indigestion<br>Kapha: loss of appetite | *A kapha type eats ice cream, resulting in the feeling of a brick in the stomach.* |
| Provocation | Increase continues, and there will likely be some discomfort in the area where the aggravated dosha is. | Vata: gas, constipation<br>Pitta: acid reflux<br>Kapha: heavy stomach, nausea | *A pitta type on a business trip enjoys too many cocktails and rich foods for an entire week, resulting in a pernicious acid stomach.* |
| Spread | The dosha begins to spill out of its site and circulate, looking for a place to reside. Signs at this level will affect daily life. | Vata: cold hands and feet, very dry skin<br>Pitta: red, irritated skin; feeling overheated<br>Kapha: congestion in sinuses, throat, or lungs | *A vata type, deep into a cold, dry winter begins to experience numbness and a lack of circulation to the extremities.* |
| Depositing | The spreading dosha sets up shop in a weak area. | The qualities of a dosha affect the function of a tissue or organ beyond its own site. | *Accumulated kapha, sticky and heavy, takes over the sinuses, resulting in a sinus infection.* |
| Manifestation | The dosha becomes strong enough to take over the weak area and affect its physical structure. | In this stage, a disorder is fully recognizable in the tissue or organ where dosha was deposited. | *The dry qualities of vata overwhelm the hip joint, weak from past injuries, and the articular surfaces dry out, break down, and vata deteriorates the joint, resulting in a hip replacement. An accumulation of the sticky qualities of kapha in an artery eventually blocks the artery and stops the flow of blood.* |
| Destruction | No longer in its early stages, disease becomes classifiable and may be giving rise to other disorders as well. | The disorder is beyond what the natural defense mechanisms of the body can handle. | *In the destruction stage, diseases are chronic or difficult to cure.* |

*Parinama*, change, is the root of aging. Essentially, we are all subject to the divine dance of time and the inescapable effects it has on the body and mind. The ancient sages realized that, although we cannot escape change, certain aspects of change are predictable. Time and the aging process have identifiable patterns and, therefore, predictable effects. The shape of a day, a season, a lifetime—these are all divisions along a continual, flowing passage of time. If we take the arc of a lifespan and break it down, we can begin to see which substances and actions promote longevity or regenerative changes and which cause degeneration. The substances we take in are food and medicine, the actions that affect us include … well, everything we do.

Ayurvedic daily and seasonal routines describe how best to flow with time over the course of a day, a season, and a life (which is why part two of the book has been organized along these lines). Working with the flow preserves health; going against it, or ignoring it, promotes disease. This wisdom was born of observing the predictable patterns of change in the environment and their effect on the body and mind.

With or without an understanding of their cosmic roots, you will find that daily and seasonal Ayurvedic routines support your health. Knowing a little about how they work and why they are important may help you home in on the routines that are most important for you.

## IN THE BLINK OF AN EYE

Time is a mind-bender. To wrap their heads around this unlimited aspect of life, Ayurveda masters subdivided the epic breadth of time into divisions to break it down into manageable durations. The smallest unit of time was the blink of an eyelid. This unit was then multiplied to create different measures, all the way up to a fortnight, a month, and a season (two months).

THE EFFECTS OF WORDS AND ACTIONS. *Karma* means "action" and implies reaction as well. An action, such as drinking turmeric milk, does not exist in a vacuum; it is part of a chain of reactions that follow, including digestion and absorption of the drink, its effect on the system, and any changes it causes. It may ground you and satisfy your appetite when you've been having a busy day, and it might keep you from doing something crazy, like eating half a box of cookies or speaking rudely to a coworker when you're hungry.

Any action begins with an impulse or desire. According to the Charaka Samhita, the enjoyment of harmful substances and activities can be a causative factor in illness. This sounds like common sense, but *prajnaparadha*—the flawed mental process where you choose things

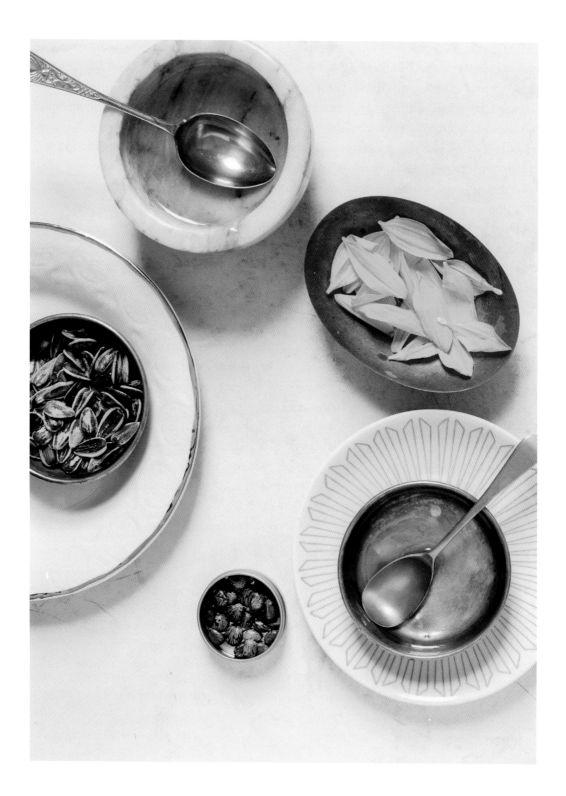

that aren't good for you, even when you know better—is the most important thing to consider about karma and the disease process. We are what we eat, do, and say. Unwholesome conduct and speech get us into trouble, so why are we drawn to unwholesome stuff?

Prajnaparadha is considered a mental imbalance. Maintaining equilibrium in the mind allows the buddhi, or intellect, to pierce through confusion and make wise choices. Self-care maintains a clear and healthy mental state. For one thing, an Ayurvedic daily routine keeps the channels of circulation open and moving and the mind clear. Think of how your mind is working (or not working) when you are congested versus after a saltwater nasal wash. Morning routines, sleep hygiene, and specific therapies such as *shiro abhyanga* (head massage with herbal oils) ensure a measured rhythm to your days, and this equilibrium reverberates in the mental sphere.

MISUSE OF THE SENSE ORGANS. The sense organs are the body parts responsible for the five senses: eyes (sight), ears (hearing), nose (smell), tongue (taste), and skin (touch). Misuse, or artha samyoga, can mean too much or too little stimulation of the senses. The nervous system is taxed by digesting too much information from the sense organs, and the organs themselves may begin to suffer. For example, your eyes become red, dry, and itchy after too much time in front of a computer or TV. Or in the case of too little stimulation, the eyes become cloudy and gunked up after oversleeping. Daily routines such as rinsing the eyes with cool water or using rose hydrosol drops can help them remain clear and bright and protect against future imbalances (see Care of the Eyes, Ears, and Nose, on page 90). Bringing the senses back into balance settles the nervous system, thereby reducing stress, which is often the cause of imbalance in the first place. For example, if people who have trouble sleeping limit their TV, smartphone, and computer time at night, they are more likely to enjoy a good night's rest.

Usually the problem lies in exposing the senses to too much stimulation. Here are a few general suggestions to reduce strain on the sense organs.

Hearing: Go easy on the tunes, and take a break sometimes. Silence works wonders. Notice the qualities of the music you choose and check in: is it appropriate for the time of day and your mental state? Music that is too upbeat may give you difficulty sleeping, while music containing angry lyrics might exacerbate your irritation.

Sight: Limit computer, smartphone, and TV time as much as possible. Track your screen activity, and notice how many minutes per day feels appropriate for you. Rest your eyes by closing them and taking a few deep breaths from time to time. If this proves difficult, try lying down with an eye pillow gently over your eyes to block out the light for a few minutes.

**Taste:** Stick to natural, less refined foods without added flavors, white sugars, or too much salt. Acclimate your taste buds to the lighter sensations of the natural world.

**Touch:** Oil your skin daily to quiet the nerve endings. Favor natural oils, such as sesame, coconut, and almond, over conventional moisturizers. Dress warmly when needed.

**Smell:** Use fewer products containing "fragrance." Reducing onion and garlic in your diet will reduce your need for deodorants.

### Disease Prevention

One who indulges daily in healthy foods and activities, who discriminates the good and bad of everything then acts wisely, who is not attached too much to the objects of the senses, who develops the habit of charity, of considering all as equal, of truthfulness, of pardoning and keeping company of good persons only, becomes free from all diseases.

*–Ashtanga Hrdayam, vol. 1, 4:36.*

At the end of the day, there are no secrets, only common sense. The ancient texts aren't generally telling us anything that wouldn't be obvious if we were paying attention. Which begs the question–are we paying attention?

The ability to discriminate the good and bad of everything, then act wisely, is easier said than done. When I began teaching public Ayurveda classes, it was always the same. A hand went up, "Are almonds good?" Then another, "Is milk bad? What about wheat?"

It depends. The answer is always, it depends: on the person, the amount, the timing, the state of the doshas. The language of Ayurveda is a way of observing the world, the body, and how they interact. For thousands of years, some information has persevered as human truth. Ayurvedic language illuminates the effects of diet and lifestyle, of time, of the roots and results of our actions, and of the relationship between the physical and subtle aspects of life. The information in this book is going to take time to digest and experience, but it provides a framework for understanding the holistic and interconnected nature of how life happens. With a little understanding and proactive self-care, health becomes an ongoing process that is enjoyable, feels good, and gives life a deeper meaning.

Drumroll, please. I give you the ancient secrets of disease prevention. Natural urges are the key! Keeping these urges a secret can get you into trouble. We have some urges that are *not* good, such as envy, greed, and sloth. But good urges arise when the body is trying to make something happen, like when hunger signals a need for food. If you eat, you maintain balance; if you suppress hunger on a regular basis, the digestive fire can get out of balance, which is a seed for a host of problems, including the formation of *ama,*

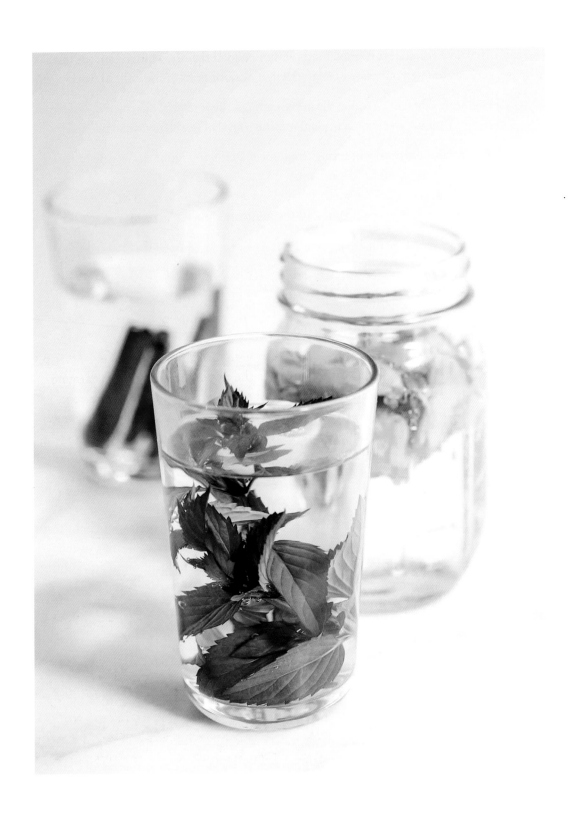

toxic sludge (more on that later). The urges described are natural and so important they are considered the key to *roganutpeedaya* (disease prevention). The essence of disease prevention includes only two rules:

1. Do not suppress natural urges.
2. Do not forcibly initiate these urges.

The body is smart and has an undeniable will to survive. There's no need to force it! The body governs the ins and outs with things like hunger and thirst (in) and burps, poop, and farts (out). Ayurveda says it is the tendency to mess with these natural processes that begins and perpetuates disease. By suppressing any of the thirteen natural urges on a regular basis, you can disrupt the flowing currents of the body that are carrying nutrition, waste, and everything else where they need to go.

I had a friend who led travel tours all over the world. What happens when you are on a bus with fifty people and you have to pee? Do you stop the bus? My friend got into the habit of holding in the pee, and after a few years, culminating with a month-long bus trip, he ended up in the hospital with a catheter because he couldn't pee. This is an extreme example, I know, but you see how the suppression of this urge disturbed the current. However, trying to push out the pee at the wrong time will also disturb the natural urge if this becomes a habit. Overcoming natural urges with mental effort catches up with you, and eventually the natural urge will become elusive. Out of the following thirteen bodily processes, I'll bet most people suppress or force at least a few sometimes, if not all the time:

| | | | |
|---|---|---|---|
| ⬩ Farts | ⬩ Thirst | ⬩ Cough | ⬩ Tears |
| ⬩ Poop | ⬩ Hunger | ⬩ Breath | ⬩ Vomit |
| ⬩ Pee | ⬩ Sleep | ⬩ Yawn | ⬩ Semen |
| ⬩ Sneeze | | | |

Texts describe the specific imbalances that can result from messing with each of these urges. The disruption of natural urges often has external and/or mental factors. There will certainly be times when these actions just have to wait. But the less this happens, the better. In many cultures, people put social codes above their own health, and the habit is contagious. It is quite common for a client's digestive imbalance to begin with a poorly digested lunch, eaten in a rush while working. When we discuss how to shift this habit, people tell me nobody at the office stops for lunch; it's simply impossible. The culture of the workplace in this example is causing digestive distress. What comes first—work culture or health? When my clients have approached a supervisor from a balanced, steady place and asked for a lunch break for the sake of their health, I have seen cooperation in every case.

I remember my first trip to India. I was blown away by the nose picking—it was absolutely fine to dig one's finger into a nostril while waiting on the bench at the train station. I couldn't believe it! This just goes to show that what we think is OK or not OK is based on social conditioning. An aspect of office culture being accepted by many does not make it right for everyone. Upon investigation, many of us might find instances where natural urges feel like an inconvenience, but what if we were taught they are heralds of health-giving habits and there is no shame in answering the call? Changing your relationship to urges, like any lifestyle change, takes time and is best approached gently. As the number-one aspect of disease prevention, it's worth it.

## PRACTICE TIP

Take another look at the list of urges, maybe in the morning before you begin your day. Have this in the back of your mind as you go through the day, and jot down in your calendar or on a sticky note if you notice yourself forcing or suppressing one of these urges. No judgment; just keep track. If you are really into it, do this for a few days or even a week. You can just make a mark next to the urge if you catch it again. Next, begin to notice if there is a certain time of day, activity, or company you are keeping that is contributing to how you are reacting to this urge. Once you see the pattern, you can begin to consider why this happens, and think about changing your flow to make time and space for natural urges. Enlisting someone you trust to support you in this change can be very helpful.

### Two Methods of Healing

Ayurveda has two branches of healing therapies: *shamana*, those that settle the doshas in the early stages of imbalance, such as oil massage and use of herbal tonics; and *shodhana*, purification therapies that remove excess doshas from the body. This might include use of laxatives, enemas, vomiting, strong nasal medications, and traditionally, bloodletting. Serious stuff! Shodhana therapies are part of the *panchakarma* process, a three- or four-week cleansing process made up of specific diet, herbs, and therapies that includes an essential preparation period and finishes with a rejuvenation period. The body is prepared by softening the channels and moving displaced doshas to the digestive tract. Nothing happens until the doshas are ripe for removal. Then a purification period begins. The rejuvenation period involves rest and rejuvenating nutrition and takes one to three months.

The removal of doshas from the body is a sensitive process, usually done at a residential center with a doctor checking in daily and deciding the next move according to what arises. This procedure can be very effective in more chronic or severe imbalances. There is no DIY good-for-everybody panchakarma program. This process should be undertaken only with experienced guidance.

Home cleansing, however, can be an excellent practice for general health, provided it is done at the right time. Ayurveda first takes into account the ratio of the strength of the person to the strength of the imbalance. A person should be strong enough to undergo cleansing. A period of cleansing should be modified according to the need for reducing or building qualities, body type, and the duties and daily schedule of the person. Without instigating any puking or pooping, simply removing diet and lifestyle factors that cause imbalance, for a period of time, is enough to calm increased doshas. Purification can simply mean getting rid of that which is not serving and making space for the body to adjust. For the first two stages of imbalance, a moderate home cleanse can keep things healthy. Some suggestions can be found in part two.

You will find lots of information and DIY shamana therapies in the daily and seasonal regimens of part two—as well as in the recipes in part three—for maintaining health by balancing qualities according to body type and season.

Now that we've explored the concept of health, disease prevention, and factors that can cause imbalance and disease, let's move into some deeper aspects of the physical, mental, senses, and soul. Next is the physical body, the tissues that build it up, the channels that move things around, and Ayurveda's number-one health factor: digestive fire.

◆

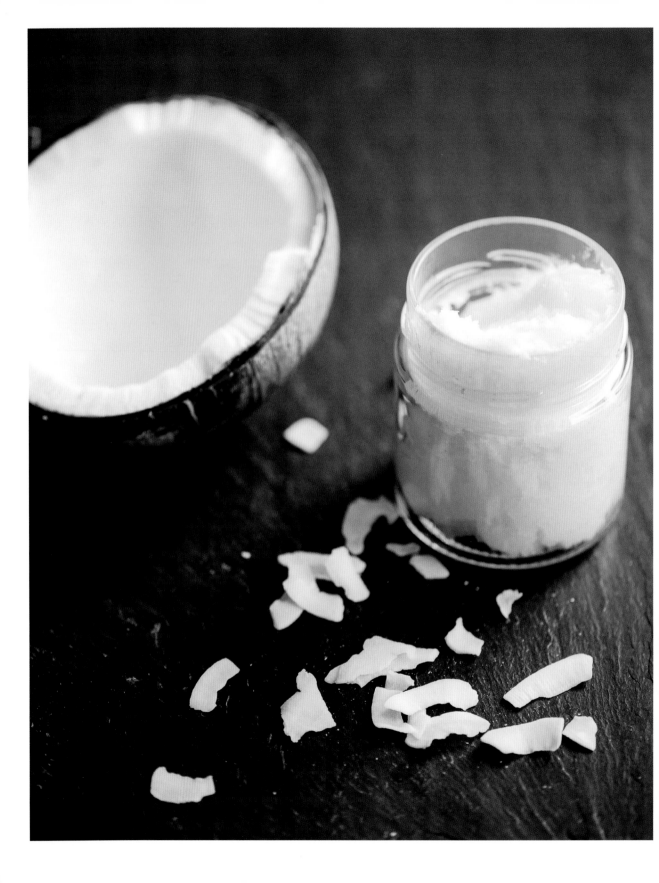

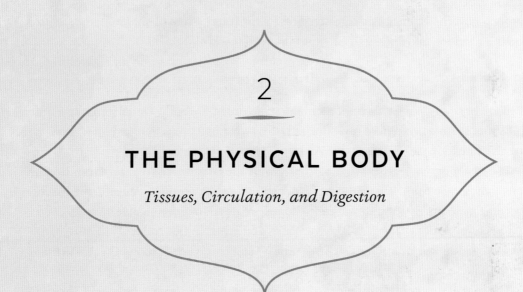

# THE PHYSICAL BODY

*Tissues, Circulation, and Digestion*

As you know by this point, the five elements make up the physical body. These elements compound into three doshas that bring their qualities and energies to the body and govern specific functions. But there's more! The physical body—substratum for the activity of the doshas, senses, and mind and container for the soul—has a specific anatomy in Ayurvedic science. The stable, structural tissues of the body, things like organs, blood, muscle, and bone, are divided into seven distinct types called dhatus. These different tissue types balance the body's structure and are nourished by a digestive process governed by agni, or digestive fire. An intricate system of channels, the *srotamsi*, carries nutrition and energy throughout the tissues and also the mind.

## DHATUS

Dhatus, or seven tissue types, maintain the structure of the body. Understanding a little bit about these seven different tissues, as well as what nourishes them and how they receive nutrition, helps to form the Ayurvedic picture of the body.

The first four tissue types are superficial, while the latter three are internal, or deep in the body, as you can see from the table on page 39. As they progress inward, the tissues become increasingly subtle. The seven dhatus are listed in order of superficial to deep. This is important because the layers are also nourished in this order. The *rasa* dhatu receives food-juice (*ahara rasa*) first, digests what it needs, sends along the rest to *rakta* dhatu, and so on.

The root of the word *dhatu* means "that which holds." The body's physicality holds its shape, while so many of its processes are dynamic, moving and transforming within that shape. The root also means "building block," and in chemistry, "base material." Each of the tissue types is made of its own kind of cells and is uniform in quality, made of a particular combination of the elements. Some of the tissues, such as fat, require heavier and denser qualities, while others, such as bone marrow, are lighter and subtle. Taking in substances that have similar qualities to a dhatu will increase it, while not taking in enough nourishing substance will cause a dhatu to decrease.

The Charaka Samhita tells us roughly the amount of each dhatu a body should have (relative to one's general size, of course).[1] The tissue types exist in relation to one another, which means if you end up with too much of one, you are then likely to have too little of another. Resources may be used up by one tissue layer, leaving another without. For example, picture an athlete who doesn't eat enough to keep up with the demands of training. The muscle layer will take all the nutrition and body fat will decrease, eventually causing a deficiency in the next layer as well, the bones.

## THE TISSUE HIERARCHY

| Dhatu | Tissue Type |
| --- | --- |
| Rasa | Plasma |
| Rakta | Red blood cells |
| Mamsa | Muscle |
| Meda | Fat |
| Asthi | Bones and cartilage |
| Majja | Bone marrow, nerve tissue, connective tissue |
| Shukra/artava | Male and female reproductive tissue, respectively |

Taking care to maintain equilibrium of the dhatus ensures a healthy state, which is why the art of balancing the five elements in the diet is so important (and why a diet of only juice or only meat is not considered a good long-term plan). There is also quite a science in Ayurvedic medicine to rectifying imbalance in the dhatus with diet and herbal remedies. A key is to introduce the qualities needed. Building tissues requires the right kind of building blocks. Certain substances have affinities for certain tissues and will create sound structure. For example, cow's milk has moist, cool, heavy qualities that, when digested well, nourish the reproductive tissue. Ghee has very unctuous, penetrating, and cooling qualities that provide a buffer for the heat produced by the constant activity of conduction in the nerve tissues and keep those tissues well lubricated. Awareness of the dhatus, and the substances that nourish each layer, can be instrumental in choosing the best foods and remedies for self-care.

## TISSUE TROUBLESHOOTING

A robust dhatu is more resistant to trouble. Unlike the doshas, which are dynamic, the dhatus are static, which makes them vulnerable to disease. Many circulating signs and symptoms can be ignored for a long time before doshas begin to damage tissues. Hence Ayurveda's focus on preventive measures and a keen awareness of early signs and symptoms. While this book isn't a be-all and end-all for understanding bodily tissues and their equilibrium, it can help you understand why a certain food or remedy might provide the qualities your tissues are craving.

## Rasa Dhatu

The word *rasa* here means "sap" or "juice." This aspect of the body is what makes a person appear and feel juicy, or full of life. You likely think of blood as red, but it is just the red blood cells that make it red; the rest is a cool, clear, unctuous liquid. This substance, called plasma, is made up of water, salts, enzymes, white blood cells, and proteins. In Ayurveda, it contains all five elements, mostly water, and its function is to nourish the body. The entire lymphatic system is made up of rasa dhatu, which makes it an important player in detoxification as well as nutrition. It is the only dhatu that circulates and penetrates the entire body. The Charaka Samhita tells us that from rasa, "the digestive product of food," is derived "continuity of strength, satisfaction, plumpness, and enthusiasm." [2]

Compromised rasa results from not eating enough, too much bitter and astringent food, dehydration, and consistent worry. It can also come from being overnourished, congested, and swollen.

Drinking enough water and keeping good circulation through moderate physical activity are two big ways to keep the rasa healthy and moving freely. Foods that are favored to nourish rasa dhatu are generally liquid, cooling, oily, and sweet, such as dates, ghee, coconut oil, almonds, soups (especially bone broth), and milk.

Yoga excels not only at increasing circulation but also at removing pranic blockages. The postures and sequencing are designed to support free movement of the vital energy throughout the body. The difference between exercise and yoga is the mind. An experienced yoga instructor teaches how to keep the breath rhythmic and cultivate the skill of moving breath through sticky parts of the body. This process begins with concentration. Where the attention goes, the prana flows, and learning how to concentrate on different areas of the body, especially the ones that are a bit murky in the beginning, creates free movement of breath and, eventually, of rasa dhatu as well.

**RECIPES FOR RASA**

Lubrication Station  204

Radiance Saffron-Almond Milk  209

Tulsi Water  173

**RECOVERING FROM BURNOUT**

The subtle transformation of food nutrients into each tissue layer takes five days, so that's thirty-five days for nutrition to reach every layer! This means if you put the pedal to the metal or don't eat enough for a while, it could take five weeks to feel you're at full power again. If you overdo the activity or underdo the nourishment for too long, sleeping in for a day just isn't going to cut it.

## Rakta Dhatu

The word *rakta* means "red." While what we usually think of as blood contains both rasa and rakta dhatus, it is the rakta that contains red blood cells, and these two parts of the blood have different compositions and functions. This tissue is made up of fire and water elements; it is hot, and its function is life-giving (*jivana*)—the oxygenation of the body by red blood cells. Planet Earth is unique because humans can breathe oxygen here, and this life breath is transported throughout the body by rakta dhatu. A healthy rakta dhatu will result in a zest for life, a rosy complexion, and a visible luster, especially to the skin and eyes.

Too much sour, spicy, and salty food, smoking, drinking too much alcohol, and iron and B vitamin deficiencies all contribute to an overheated or deficient, unhealthy rakta.

Adequate relaxation time, noncompetitive and moderate exercise, and a diet that includes sweet, cooling, and red-colored foods like red grapes, pomegranate, blueberries, ripe cherries, plums, and beets, as well as bitter green vegetables, will optimize the health of this dhatu.

**RECIPES FOR RAKTA**

Cardamom-Ginger Grape Elixir  253
Spicy Dandelion Green Soup  224
Aloe Pomegranate Cooler  179
Cooling Neem Massage Oil  250

## Mamsa Dhatu

Earth and water elements provide the heavy and dense qualities necessary to create muscle tissue. In Ayurveda, the function of muscle is *lepana*, or plastering, which means holding the skeleton together, in the same way you would plaster a wall to further stabilize the frame. The subtissue of *mamsa* dhatu is composed of the underlying layers of skin (not the outermost, which is a subtissue of rasa) and subcutaneous fat. When the mamsa dhatu is weak, a person will appear sunken and lack self-confidence. A healthy mamsa will yield strength in both body and mind.

Too much exercise, too much sweating, stress, lack of sleep, and too much light food or too much heavy food can all contribute to an unhealthy mamsa dhatu.

The right amount of protein, sleep, and weight-bearing exercise ensure a healthy mamsa. More is not necessarily better.

**RECIPES FOR MAMSA**

Ashwagandha Ghee  242
Bone Builder  207
Ayur-Evening Treat  207

## Meda Dhatu

Earth and water provide the structure for fat, or adipose, tissue, which is heavy, slimy, and dense. The primary function of this tissue is lubrication, and *meda* dhatu is responsible for its subtissues, tendons, sinews, and ligaments. Without enough of meda's lubricating qualities, these connective tissues will dry out, as will the skin and eventually the bones. For example, excessive exercise can cause so much nutrition to go to the muscle layer that meda, the next in line for nourishment, gets the short end of the stick.

Having too much fat will cause an excess of heavy quality that can result in lethargy, stagnation, and congestion. The right amount of fat tissue brings a feeling of comfort, protects against cold and dry qualities, and, according to the classical texts, results in "beauty," which is not only a physical thing in this context. Abundance is beautiful.

Too much or too little food or exercise, as well as a low digestive fire (discussed later in this chapter) or metabolism, can result in the wrong amount of meda dhatu. Stress can be indirectly responsible when it causes under- or overeating and disturbs the digestive fire. Indigestible fats that are denatured (hydrogenated, fractionated), as well as old and rancid oils, can cause toxicity in the meda dhatu.

Taking care to balance building foods with smaller amounts of bitter, pungent foods in the diet will ensure the body can break down heavier foods nicely. Pungent substances are especially helpful in burning through extra fat in a meal and in the body. Try using the agni-boosting recipes, especially in damp, cool weather. This environment has moist, dense qualities like fat tissue. A gentle cleanse from time to time is also an excellent way to keep this dhatu in balance.

**RECIPES FOR MEDA**

Pepper-Honey Fat Burner 185
Spicy Hot Honey 198
Ajwain Water 168

## Asthi Dhatu

Bone tissue is made up of predominantly earth element and is very mineral dense. Bones are porous and hollow, however, so the space element is also present. The function of bone tissue is support (*dharana*). The articular cartilage in the joints is affected by the health of *asthi* dhatu, while teeth, hair, and nails are secondary tissues of the bone layer and can tell a story about how the bones are doing. If teeth, hair, or nails become brittle, the gums are receding, or the hair is falling out, then it is likely the asthi dhatu is compromised. Joint pain and cracking in the joints can also be a sign. Too much bone tissue is much less common than too little, but it can cause bone spurs and calcification.

**RECIPES FOR ASTHI**

Bone Builder  207

Juicy Joints Hemp Milk  210

Basic Cured Sesame Oil  245

The tissue that supports the shape of the body and protects the vital organs is the first of the deep tissues. When the body is not receiving proper nourishment, it is in these layers that imbalances first become apparent, as they are the farthest from the circulating rasa. Deficiency in any of the deep tissues can cause sensations of insecurity, fear, weakness, and lack of energy.

Leading a lifestyle that overtaxes the mind, being continually on the run, multitasking, and stressing out increase stress hormones that draw the prana to circulate more in the external tissues. A concentration or meditation practice is a great way to steady the attention inward and invite nourishment into the bone tissue.

Including mineral-rich foods in the diet helps to keep asthi dhatu robust. Seeds and seaweeds both are very concentrated mineral sources. Sesame seeds and sesame oil are traditionally favored for all of the deep tissues, as they contain a bit of pungency that helps the good fats penetrate to the deeper layers. In addition to seeds of all sorts, milk, green vegetables, and legumes are other good foods for asthi. Bone broths and meat stews are mentioned in the classics as medicine for deficiency.

*Dharana*, the sixth limb of Patanjali's yoga system, means "concentration," or the ability to hold the attention on one point. This skill is considered a prerequisite to meditation. It seems no accident that the same word is used to describe the supporting function of the bones. The unwavering, concentrated energy of earth element in the bones is like the quality of mind experienced in dharana. Concentrating on the quality of the skeleton, especially in standing postures where it is bearing weight, will strengthen not only the bones but also the mind.

## Majja Dhatu

*Majja* dhatu is the nerve tissue of the body, and its function is *purana*, "to fill space." The space in the bones contains bone marrow, which is majja dhatu. This jelly-like substance is liquid and oily and supports the bone. Not enough jelly and the bones will be weak.

### RECIPES FOR MAJJA

Brahmi Ghee  239
Jar o' Ojas  215
Stress-Be-Gone Tonic  206
Stress-Ease Brahmi Oil  249

Majja dhatu is also responsible for conduction, or the intercellular communication that moves through the nerves. In this way, nerve tissue fills the space between cells and systems by creating communication. Nerve tissue carries sensory input (sensation), determines motor function, and transmits information via microscopic fibers called neurotransmitters. The majja dhatu makes up a subtle communication line that goes throughout the body. The secretions of the eyes are a subtissue, including tears. When majja is healthy, perception is clear, the eyes are bright, and the mind is sharp and steady. Problems in the majja dhatu occur due to any of the doshas acting on it and can cause disorders such as shingles, sciatica, and insomnia.

Long-term or extreme stress, trauma, and chronic undernourishment can lead to an imbalance in the nerve tissue layer.

Ghee is revered for its ability to penetrate and rejuvenate nerve tissue with its moist, oily, and slightly cool nature. Nerve activity creates heat, and my yoga teacher would always recommend ghee in the diet to balance the heating effect that certain practices can have on the nerves. Coconut oil is second only to ghee. Keeping enough moisture in the body is key. Traditionally, targeted, herbal ghee-based nerve tonics called *ghritas* were used for rejuvenation of the majja dhatu.

## Shukra and Artava Dhatus

*Shukra* and *artava* are the male and female reproductive tissues, respectively. Their function is fertility and reproduction. Both are liquid and unctuous and, like the nerve tissue, are rejuvenated by cooling substances. The sperm, egg, ovaries, testes, and their lubrication are all included in this tissue layer. *Ojas*, the nutrient cream of the body, is the end product of all tissue nutrition and is considered a secondary tissue of the reproductive system. Most substances that build ojas are also aphrodisiacs, because they increase fertility and nourish reproductive tissues.

Too much spicy food and drying, heating foods such as alcohol and coffee can compromise this tissue. Too much sex, preoccupation with sex, too much stress, and a diet predominant in pungent, bitter, and/or astringent tastes can cause disorders in this dhatu and contribute to infertility. For women, overworking or overexercising during the menstrual cycle can compromise the artava dhatu.

**RECIPES FOR SHUKRA/ARTAVA**

Shatavari Ghee 241

Ashwagandha Ghee 242

Radiance Saffron-Almond Milk 209

Lubrication Station 204

Maintaining a conscious and loving sex life is the best medicine for this tissue, where overdoing it or repressing it both can cause problems. Rejuvenate with sweet and oily foods gently spiced with ginger, cinnamon, and saffron, especially dates, soaked almonds, walnuts, sesame, and hemp. For men, ashwagandha is known for increasing vitality and libido, while for women, shatavari's cool, soft qualities are favored.

Balanced dhatus are one of the hallmarks of swastha, a healthy person. As they exist in relationship to one another, maintaining their balance is generally achieved through a well-rounded, seasonal diet and the right amount of exercise. Throughout an annual cycle, Ayurvedic knowledge suggests a rotating cast of the six tastes, which bring all of the elements into the body at the right time.

## Upadhatus and Malas

The tissues also have sub-, or secondary, tissues called *upadhatus*. These minitypes have very specific functions and do not act as building blocks like the dhatus do, so they are considered subtissues. The state of a subtissue can show whether or not its dhatu is in good shape. Examples include the top layer of skin, menstrual blood, tendons, and teeth.

Mala is waste, "that which needs to be secreted from the body," comprising impurities that result from the metabolic activity in the tissue. Anytime digestion happens, there is likely to be a little waste product, and dhatu mala is how each tissue gets rid of waste. These are fun things like urine, poop, and sweat.

## THE BODY AND SROTAMSI

We know that in the workings of the body, a lot of stuff gets moved around. Fluids, wastes, nutritive materials, and energy, to name a few, are constantly being transported throughout the body by an intricate system of tubes. These tubes are called *srotamsi* in Ayurveda, and a single tube is called a *srotas*. The word suggests the activity of flowing, and this channel system is constantly in a state of flow. The subtle and gross pathways circulate throughout the entire body, including the dhatus. Each pathway has a beginning, an end, and a passage in between.

The channels referred to can be obvious and physical, as well as subtle and invisible to the eye. The *mahasrotas*, or biggest channel, is the digestive tract. Ayurveda considers the healthy function of this channel to be of the utmost importance. Other physical channels include, for example, those that carry sweat and urine out of the body and through which the muscle and fatty tissues are built. The skin contains innumerable pores, each one a channel that releases sweat. Subtle channels include nerves and tiny capillaries.

Such channels can get gunked up and eventually clogged by plaque, or ama, and cause stagnation. Clogged arteries are a great example. They can also become misshapen, shrunken, or swollen (as in the case of inflammation), which can impede the passage, or the pace, of movement through the channel. In extreme cases, a channel can rupture and the wrong thing can end up in the wrong place. Take heart, because many of the self-care practices, bodywork, and dietary wisdom of Ayurveda work behind the scenes to maintain healthy channels. Often yoga postures, breathing techniques, and visualizations are also designed to increase circulation and break up energetic blockages.

What is so absolutely cool about the srotamsi is that Ayurveda and yoga texts also point toward an extremely subtle and at times mystical set of channels through which prana, or energy, travels throughout the body. These internal channels include the moving energy of the senses, such as the eyes and ears, a channel for the movements of the mind, and an infinite number of invisible passages, called *nadis*, for the circulation of prana. The entire body is connected through a subtle circulatory network–physically, mentally, and energetically.

Learning about the channel system of the body helps us to understand the nature of the living body, its connectivity, and the importance of circulation. To visualize this network of passages and the immeasurable movements occurring at all times brings a dynamic sense of how things work. Keeping the channels healthy and the energy moving is an indispensable aspect of health. While you might think it's your shoulder you are working on, it may be something much deeper, and your self-care efforts can affect an

## CIRCULATION STATION

If the image of clogged channels inspires you to exercise, you are on the right track! Exercise is the best medicine for keeping the circulation going and the channels clear. Consider the Ayurvedic routine of exercising in the morning on an empty stomach. Getting your heat up by moving the body increases the fire element. It is this fire that spreads and burns the plaque that clogs channels. If you haven't eaten anything yet, your exercise efforts can go directly toward burning up anything your body wasn't able to metabolize during the night.

Practice tip: If you are used to eating first thing, it can take a little time to adjust to exercising on an empty stomach. Begin by eating just a little something—I find a Medjool date or other sweet fruit, or a teaspoon of nut butter, works well. At first, I ate too much and then too little, until I figured out that for me, one date was the way to go. I needed that sometimes. Now that my digestion is accustomed to eating after exercise, it's never a problem. Keep in mind that in cases of hypoglycemia or acid stomach, a different flow may be in order, and you might consult a practitioner about the best morning routine for you. Remember that exercise at any time of day is beneficial.

entire circulatory network, freeing up energy that can heal other parts of you, which may not have seemed interconnected. In this way, activities and remedies that increase circulation in general are at the root of self-care in Ayurvedic medicine.

While there are tens of thousands of channels, Ayurvedic medicine notes thirteen principal internal channels, nine external ones, and a channel for the mind.[3] An external channel opens to the outside of the body, while internal channels generally travel within. The classical texts are purposely a little vague and suggest that a true understanding of the channel system of the body requires wisdom born of practice.

In modern times, these thirteen internal channels are taught with more detail to Ayurveda students. Each channel has a place, or places, where it originates in the body, a definite pathway, and an opening, which is an important spot for administering healing therapies. For our purposes, try to visualize these channels in your body. It can help in understanding some of the interconnections going on in there, as well as a little bit about the ins and outs of the body. Of these channels, three bring stuff into the body, three take waste out of the body, and seven nourish the seven tissue layers.

## Channels for Food, Prana, and Water

The food channel, or *annavahasrotas*, begins in the esophagus and stomach and travels through the digestive tract, ending at the ileocecal valve, where the small intestine ends and the large intestine begins. It is in this channel that food is broken down into a nutrient liquid and the assimilation of the nutrients into the body from the small intestine occurs. Chewing well is important so the food ingested goes into the esophagus smoothly and is broken down completely in the stomach.

The *pranavahasrotas* brings life energy into the body. This channel is seated in the heart, travels through the respiratory tract, and ends at the nose. Breathing exercises, specifically the nasal breathing encouraged in yoga practice, are a direct line to the channel of prana. Breathing through the mouth will not have the same effect. Free breathing oxygenates and invigorates all the cells of the body. There's a fountain of youth right there!

The channel that carries water into the body is called *ambuvahasrotas*. This channel begins with the pancreas, where the blood sugar is regulated, and the secretions of cerebrospinal fluid in the brain. The soft palate (the roof of the mouth) is connected to the place in the brain where this fluid is secreted. The passage of the water channel is the mucous membrane of the entire gastrointestinal tract. The openings of the channel are the kidneys, the tongue, and the sweat glands. So, you can see that water is everywhere! Ambuvahasrotas is circulating water element through the body in the digestive system, the blood, the brain, and spinal cord and all of the body's mucous membranes.

### THE SEAT OF PRANA IS IN THE HEART

Whether the ancients meant the spiritual heart or the physical heart is up for debate even today. The organ of the heart is certainly an important player, but why does our "heart" hurt when we are sad? Why do we feel emotional pain in the chest area? Where does the phrase "a broken heart" come from? It seems there is, and always has been, a connection between the two realities of heart, physical and subtle, which can't be ignored. Perhaps the message for us in modern times is to pay equal attention to care of physical heart health and spiritual health. It seems quite obvious to me, when I am working with a person who is brokenhearted, that healing needs to occur for the inner self in order to get lasting results for the body at large. *Sneha*, which means both "love" and "oil" and is a Sanskrit word used for oil massage, is an excellent home therapy for this kind of healing.

Too much or too little water, or abnormality in its circulation, can take many shapes. For a simple example, consider too little water in the mucous membranes and how that might show up. Dry nose? Dry poops? Dry mouth? Or consider too much water. Swelling? Excess mucus? Feeling gunked up in the gut? Something like oil pulling (see chapter 5) can access the channel via the tongue and soft palate, increasing circulation and bringing moisture throughout, while breaking a sweat can remove some water via the sweat glands.

## The Channels for Eliminating

Getting rid of wastes is a huge part of being healthy, as the body will reabsorb toxins that are unable to exit through these eliminatory channels. As mentioned in chapter 1, one of the ways we get in trouble is by suppressing the urge to poop or pee, which can cause distress in the channel in the long run. If something is trying to move down and out and it gets squeezed back in, eventually the down-and-out pattern weakens, and elimination suffers. Suppressing sweat by wearing antiperspirant is also ill-advised. The good news is that a clean body doesn't stink much, even when sweating.

There are three channels for the three malas (poop, pee, and sweat). The channel that carries and eliminates feces is called *purishavahasrotas*. The cecum, which connects the small to the large intestine, is where this channel begins. Poop travels through the entire large intestine and rectum, and the opening of the channel is the anus.

*Mutravahasrotas* carries urine out of the body. The root of the channel is the kidneys, where wastewater is processed out of the blood and sent from the kidneys down the ureters to the bladder, the passageway of the channel. The opening is the urethra, or pee hole, to be scientific.

The channel that carries sweat is called *svedavahasrotas*. It begins in the sweat glands, travels through the sweat ducts, and opens at the pores of the skin. Since it is opening at the skin, health of the sweat channel is closely related to the health of the skin. The skin, being infinitely porous, is our largest sensory organ and provides a bodywide passageway between the internal and external channels of the body.

## The Channels Nourishing the Seven Tissue Layers

Between the ins and outs is the nutrition of the tissues. These seven channels, the dhatu srotamsi, correspond to the seven tissue layers: lymph and plasma, red blood cells, muscle, fat, bone, nerve tissue, and reproductive tissue. If one of these channels were to become blocked or inflamed, or move too fast or too slow, the tissue that it nourishes would suffer, as well as all of the ones that come after it.

1. *Rasavahasrotas,* the channel that carries plasma, is rooted in the heart and the "ten great vessels." [4] These vessels are subtle channels that emanate from the heart and carry ojas, which supports the body's life force and immunity. [5] The channel passes through the veins and arteries and opens at the capillaries where they meet. Ojas, an unctuous, nutritive liquid, permeates the entire body and is the basis of all the tissue nutrition that follows. The root of the channel is in the heart, suggesting there is a strong energetic component to this channel. Think of it as circulating not only nutritive juice but also life energy, and a full spiritual heart plays a part in feeling juicy.

2. *Raktavahasrotas,* the channel that carries blood, is rooted in the liver and spleen, travels through the arterial circulatory system, and, like rasa, opens at the capillaries where veins and arteries meet. This channel also draws from the red bone marrow, which, like blood, has a red hue and produces red blood cells. Foods that are red are considered blood builders, especially pomegranate, red grapes, and beets.

3. *Mamsavahasrotas,* the channel that nourishes the muscle, is rooted in the fascia, small tendons, and skin. It travels through the muscular system and opens at the skin. Oil massage is a great therapy for this layer, as it increases circulation in the skin and the connective tissue just beneath it. In the case of dryness, pain, and muscle wasting or weakness, a rich and warming oil like sesame is indicated. In the case of excessive heat or burning soreness, an oil that calms heat and inflammation such as coconut or castor can be used. (Find more information on oil massage and its uses in chapter 8.)

4. *Medavahasrotas,* the channel that nourishes the fat tissue, is rooted in the omentum and the adrenals; it passes through subcutaneous fat (the roughly half-inch layer just under the skin) and opens at the sweat glands. This is why sweating is so good for detoxifying, as the fat tissue tends to be a place where toxins are stored. Keep in mind it's better to sweat a little bit most days than going full-on every now and then.

5. *Asthivahasrotas,* the channel that nourishes the bone, is rooted in the pelvis and sacrum, travels through the skeletal system, and opens at the nails and hair. If the nails and hair become brittle, this can be a heads-up that bone health is suffering. Standing desks, walking, and standing yoga postures that load the weight evenly through the pelvis—such as Tree Pose (Vriksasana) and the Warrior Poses (Virabhadrasana)—circulate energy through the root of this channel and can be helpful for bone density.

6. *Majjavahasrotas,* the channel for the nerve tissue, is rooted in the brain and spinal cord and the joints. It passes through the entire nervous system, and opens in the space between nerves, or the synaptic space. This channel is also responsible for tears. Communication must continue to flow through this channel for the nervous system to operate effectively. Ayurveda often recommends herbal ghees to lubricate the channel, keeping the nerve tissues moist and responsive.

7. *Shukra/artavavahasrotas,* the channel for nourishment of the reproductive tissue, is rooted in the testicles, ovaries, and nipples, and passes through all of the reproductive organs. It opens for the male in the urethra; for women, it opens in the vagina. Observing and respecting the cyclical nature of the reproductive system is helpful in ensuring good circulation. At times, the body is asking to slow down and bring the focus to the deep channels, when too much activity can continue to circulate the energy outward. Generally, around the new moon is the best time to quiet down and turn the attention inward. Around the full moon, it may feel natural to be more social and get out and about.

### The Channel of the Mind

*Manovahasrotas,* the channel of the mind, remains a bit esoteric and is not expounded upon much by Ayurveda texts, though yogic texts deal greatly with the mind and nadis, or subtle channels. It is understood that yogis were the specialists in this area, and while the health of the mind and the body are impossible to separate, the Ayurvedic physician might refer out to a yoga specialist in cases where the channel of the mind is greatly afflicted. The seat of this channel is the heart, more likely the spiritual heart, or the place of prana, than the physical organ of the heart. The channel of the mind is said to pulsate throughout the entire body. [6] The pervasive nature of the mind is an important point. The mind in an overwhelmed state can circulate stress throughout the entire body. Likewise, efforts to maintain a healthy spiritual life and feed the soul circulate subtle nutrients and healing energy throughout the body. "Mind over matter" takes on a new significance when viewed as an active part of the channel system of the body.

The channel of the mind is one of those aspects of the body that can't be seen or measured by physical instruments. The mind can be sensed or felt. There are, in fact, many parts of humans that can't be seen by the naked eye. Our life energy, our breath, our mental processes, our digestive fire–although they are invisible, these are undoubtedly important aspects of health. What makes Ayurveda so illuminating is the equal emphasis it places on the four aspects of life: body, mind, senses, and soul.

# AGNI

Agni is the fire element, and fire manifests in human beings as the spark of life. It is the spark of hunger that renders food into bioavailable nutrition, the spark of the intelligence that navigates us through the world, and the subtle metabolic factors deep within the body. Agni is the most important factor of health. It is responsible for all nutrition, as well as for burning away impurities.

All of the agni in the body is governed by the main fire, *jathara agni*, the digestive fire, which resides in the lower part of the stomach. If the jathara agni is out of balance, slowing down, flaring up, or irregular, all of the agni in the body will eventually become affected. Think of jathara agni as the command center for all digestive and metabolic activity.

Caring for the digestive fire in the stomach is the easiest way to preserve health. A strong agni will ensure that the tissues are nourished and that nothing that isn't supposed to be there is able to survive, anywhere in the body. Strong agni cooks away impurities. Weak agni allows for poorly digested food to sit around in the stomach, which over time begins to congeal into a thick, sticky sludge that is very hard to get rid of. This substance, called ama, stays in the stomach initially and sits upon the agni, dampening the fires of digestion, which makes production of more ama likely. A catch-22! Over time, ama can also end up in other places in the body. It is the building block of disease and creates fatigue, body aches, brain fog, poor appetite, and a bad smell in the mouth, sweat, and feces. Ama in the stomach can be spotted as a thick, opaque coating on the back of the tongue that does not scrape off.

Taking care of the agni in the stomach is like watching over a campfire. The right amount of logs and kindling are offered into the fire as it grows weaker. Fuel the fire too much, too little, too often, or not often enough and it will not burn as well or as long. Likewise, blowing on the fire gently and smoothly helps it to grow, while blowing too much or erratically will disturb the glow. The air element is present in movement, and the speed at which we eat—sitting down to eat, breathing, and relaxing—all protect the fire, whereas eating on the run, during intense conversations, or when emotional can disturb the fire. All of the Ayurvedic routines about food and mealtimes are about caring for agni. A person is as old as their agni in Ayurveda. Preserving the natural fire of appetite preserves longevity.

Feeling for the campfire in the belly is a great starting place. Get to know your appetite, pay attention to its comings and goings. Take care to eat enough to carry you to the next meal, without feeling stuffed. Take care not to ignore the appetite, and enjoy nourishment when you are hungry. Eat your largest meal around midday when the fire principle is strongest, because the sun is high. Understanding agni puts all of these Ayurvedic lifestyle

## CARE OF THE FIVE ELEMENTS IN DIGESTION

**Space**: The stomach should have some space left for the contents to move around. Leave it a quarter empty.

**Air**: Be wary of walking and talking while eating. These activities can increase air going in with the food and distract energy from the digestive process. Do not suppress burps, and stop eating once you have a burp.

**Fire**: Do not eat unless you are hungry! Make sure to eat within an hour or so of strong appetite arising so it doesn't pass you by.

**Water**: The right amount of water is important. Avoid drinking more than 8 ounces half an hour before, during, or soon after meals. Favor foods that contain moisture, such as soups and stews, which are more readily converted to food-juice.

**Earth**: Balance the density of your meals to ensure that you feel satisfied. A salad with no fat or a steak with no greens can leave you wanting.

tips and agni-boosting digestive remedies into context. If you consider how agni works in the body, get to know the feeling of strong, weak, or irregular agni, and make connections to observe how this happens, you can identify food habits or timing that may be contributing to your feeling not so great. Shift your habits, build your agni for a while with some of the agni-boosting recipes in chapter 10, and you can balance your own digestive fire.

## Four Types of Agni

The doshas can affect agni when they are imbalanced, causing four different states of agni: balanced, irregular, too sharp, and too slow. A person of any prakriti can experience any of these types of agni, but the qualities present in the body to begin with can make one type more likely. The cold quality of vata can decrease agni, while the erratic, mobile quality causes irregularity of appetite. The hot, sharp qualities of pitta can cause agni to burn too intensely. The cool, slow, dense qualities of kapha can dull the digestive fire. The strength and quality of agni are responsible for the state of the ahara rasa, the juice of food nutrients that is created in the stomach and small intestine. This nutritive fluid circulates in the body, nourishing all of the tissues. If this food-juice is not optimal, the physical tissues are compromised, and the channels that carry the ahara rasa around the body can become clogged by poor-quality juice.

The four types of agni are as follows:

1. **Sama** (balanced) agni occurs when a person's doshas are all in their relative states of balance, and the appetite is rhythmic and predictable. Generally, a square meal digests well, elimination is regular, and there is little wind or acidity to complain of. The metabolism will be good, and the skin and eyes glow. A person of any prakriti can enjoy balanced agni, though it may come easier for some than others.

2. **Vishama** (irregular) agni results from aggravated vata. The appetite will be inconsistent and may arise and leave quickly without any reason. This kind of fire can undercook or overcook food, as well as leave it in partial states of digestion. This type of ahara rasa will create gas and bloating and irregular elimination.

3. **Tikshna** (sharp) agni results from aggravated pitta. The appetite will flare up quickly and can be insatiable or even constant. Large amounts of food will still leave this person feeling unsatisfied, physically and mentally. Hypermetabolism can cause deficiency in the body. There is often some degree of pain, nausea, or acid stomach and dryness of the lips, throat, and mouth after eating.

4. **Manda** (slow, dull) agni results from aggravated kapha. The appetite is sluggish, as is the metabolism and elimination. This person may rarely feel truly hungry. Food will sit in the stomach for a long time and feel heavy. Over time, manda agni leads to undigested food sticking around in the body causing fatigue, allergies, congestion, and sadness. There will be less zest for life.

### Ama Alert

Imbalanced states of agni can lead to ama. Unchecked in the stomach, ama travels and lodges in a weak spot. It also clogs channels, blocks flow of circulation, and leads to stagnation. Think of how cholesterol, thick and sticky, compromises the flow of blood and eventually the function of the pumping heart itself. It all began with goop getting

---

**PRACTICE TIPS TO BALANCE AGNI**

**Vishama agni:** Eat simply. One-pot hot meals, soups, and stews will be ideal.

**Tikshna agni:** Slow down, sit down. Eat dense, high-calorie foods. Relax the body to receive the nutrition; paying attention to the meal increases the life energy it gives you.

**Manda agni:** Exercise on an empty stomach. Skip dinner.

stuck along the channels. Ama acts like this anyplace in the body where it hangs around. Luckily, Ayurveda texts describe clearly how ama happens and how to get rid of it.

There are only four causes to consider:

1. Imbalanced agni.
2. Stagnation of wastes: urine, poop, and sweat (think antiperspirant or creams that block the pores and the suppression of urges).
3. Doshas lodging in tissues (manage them early on to avoid this).
4. Unresolved emotions and experiences. While mental stagnation does not directly result in the physical substance ama, afflictions of the mind can promote physical stagnations that lead to the formation of ama. Imagine how your appetite becomes during extreme stress—likely one of the imbalanced states already mentioned. If that stress is not addressed, the imbalance becomes chronic.

Keep in mind that these causes take some time to develop. The body can handle a little stress or some poorly digested food from time to time. If you really want that tub of popcorn at the movie, enjoy it (and head in there with room in your stomach), but take care not to have it again tomorrow. It's when poor habits become the norm that things can get serious.

### AMA CHECKLIST

If you *consistently* experience several of the following, you might have ama. But fear not, we have a plan.

- Opaque, white coating on the tongue that doesn't scrape off
- Heavy feeling in the stomach and/or the back of the throat
- Bad taste in the mouth, bad breath
- Chronic congestion
- Grogginess after meals
- Heavy, sticky, stinky stools
- Strong body odor (more than your usual)
- Lymphatic congestion (such as swollen breasts before periods or bloating after meals)
- Constipation and/or diarrhea
- Low libido and low energy
- Mental confusion (brain fog, especially after eating)

## Build the Fire, Burn the Sludge

Protecting the digestive fire with healthy food habits is the first way to go. A strong agni will not allow ama to hang around. Ahara, an aspect of the Ayurvedic daily regimen, suggests general guidelines about how and when we should eat (see chapter 5). In the event that ama has formed, measures can be taken to "burn" it. Building agni and burning ama go hand in hand. Imagine a campfire with a sticky, slimy substance sitting in it. Kindling will be the key, added to the start of the fire and then at regular intervals to keep it burning stronger than the heavy, sticky qualities sitting in it. This kindling of the digestive fire with spices is called *deepana*. Maybe we also shoot some lighter fluid or other penetrating substance on there that will help break up the sludge. Spices that improve the quality of digestion and process ama are called *pachana*.

Most spices that kindle agni also digest ama, and it is how they are used that decides their efficacy. In general, adding kindling to the fire will also support a completely digested end product, with fewer by-products such as gas and hyperacidity. Deepana and pachana spices are also used in herbal remedies to increase the digestion of the herb and its carrier substance (such as milk or ghee) and to push the medicines deeper into the body with sharp and penetrating qualities. Now you know why certain spices are in so many of the home remedies.

Deepana spices are taken in small amounts *before food*, with a waiting period to allow the fire to grow before eating. These spices will increase the appetite. Some examples are pepper, cinnamon, cumin, mustard seed, ajwain, hing, and turmeric.

Pachana spices can be used *during* the cooking process and also taken in larger amounts *after meals* to improve digestion and absorption—especially useful after large or rich meals. Some examples are ginger, garlic, lemon, chilies, coriander, fennel, cardamom, rosemary, and thyme.

Ideally, a healthy lifestyle and diet will balance the agni, and doing damage control with spices isn't necessary all of the time. Feeding the fire in a consistent way is key. Eating too much at one

### NOTEWORTHY DEEPANA RECIPES

Fire Up the Agni Tea  186

Ginger Blaster  231

Pepper-Honey Fat Burner  185

Takra  226

### NOTEWORTHY PACHANA RECIPES

Cumin-Coriander-Fennel Tea  183

After-Meal Chewing Spice Mix  232

Appetite-Boosting Ginger Pickle  229

Dr. Claudia's Agni Soup  222

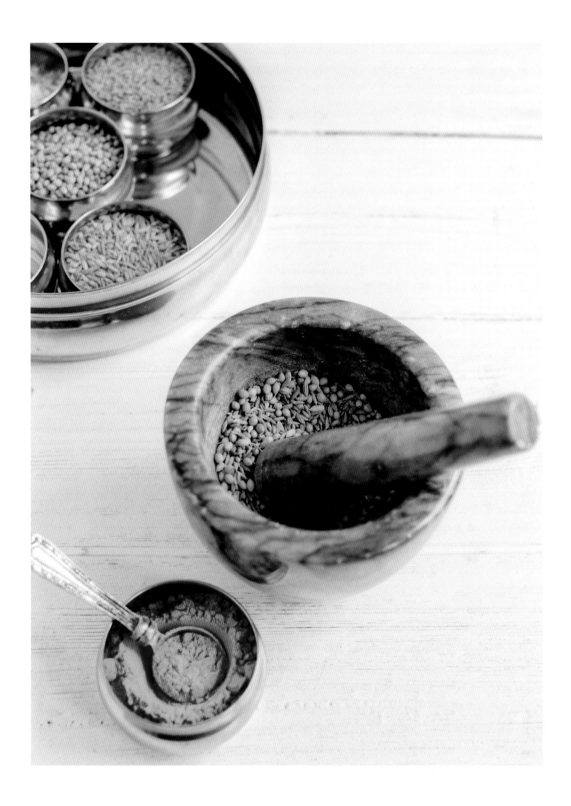

sitting really does the agni in. Ignoring hunger and letting it go so long that the appetite goes away is not helpful either. Binge eating is a setup, as are snacking and grazing, while enjoying moderate meals on a consistent schedule is the Ayurvedic way. Some people need three meals daily, some only two. Space them out by four to six hours, and allow the agni to do its job in between. This can take up to six months to adjust to.

It's easy to get used to eating too often. The ideal in Ayurveda, however, is for the agni to have some time between meals to grow and to fully process the previous foods. Healthy fats included in meals feed the agni in the same way an oil lamp burns clean and clear with good fuel. It is common for those who are used to eating often to have a hard time allowing the agni to grow to optimum between meals; the body loses the skill. Fat burning will happen between meals, usually when they are spaced out by more than four hours. To remind your body how to burn fat, slowly adopt the habit of not eating between meals. Don't rush it, as you may get hungry sooner in the beginning. It can take about six months to adjust. I see people mourn the loss of snacking in the beginning, but they soon adapt and feel more even-keeled and relaxed burning good fuel.

### Feeding All of You

Once the food-juice is created in the stomach, more subtle processes of metabolism and absorption continue, bringing the nutrition of ahara rasa to the dhatus. There are three ways this can happen. Each dhatu has its own mini-agni, which transforms nutrition into tissue. The process known as the "law of irrigation" describes the nutrient fluid circulating through the body via the rasa dhatu, the blood plasma. In the way a field is first irrigated closest to the water source and then flowing to the next section, nutrition enters rasa dhatu first, then the red blood (rakta), muscle, fat, bones, nerves, and last, the reproductive tissues. The tissues farthest from the circulating rasa receive nutrition last. If it is all used up, tissues in need of nutrition may select what they need from the rasa in the way pigeons peck at a scattering of seeds. This is called the "law of selectivity." In the "law of transformation," each dhatu is formed directly from the leftovers of the previous tissue layer and transformed by the dhatu agni of that layer. For instance, when there is not enough fat, the bones suffer because the previous dhatu used up the nutrition. There are no leftovers to transform into bone tissue.

Each of these metabolic processes nourishes the body in different ways. In the law of irrigation, it takes about one day for each dhatu to receive nourishment, so a week total. While the law of selectivity can yield nutrition faster, it is a less sustainable method, which the body resorts to in times of need. The law of transformation takes longer but results in ojas after about one month. Ojas is the final digestive product, the nutrient cream of the body, and is responsible for immunity and inner strength. Ojas is created from the nutrients remaining in the rasa after all tissues have been reached. The more ojas is produced by a nourishing diet in conjunction with strong agni, the stronger and healthier a person will be. This is why the rejuvenation period after cleansing is at least one month long—it takes that much time for all of the dhatus to be refreshed.

It helps to understand the time line of the nutrition process; in a world where things are often happening fast, feeling better can take a little time. Consider the job agni has to provide the mother fire in the gut and all the little fires throughout the tissues of the body transforming, nourishing, cleansing. It's inspiration to sit down for a quiet meal, isn't it?

Our discussion in this chapter makes up a complete picture of the body and how its parts are interconnected. Now you can really understand the Ayurvedic definition of health! If health is a state of balanced doshas, agni, and dhatus, normal removal of wastes, and pleasant mind, senses, and soul, we are getting close to seeing the whole picture. Now that you know how doshas and agni work, how the tissues are maintained, and how wastes get moved out of the body, let's move on to the subtle body, where we find the mind, senses, and soul.

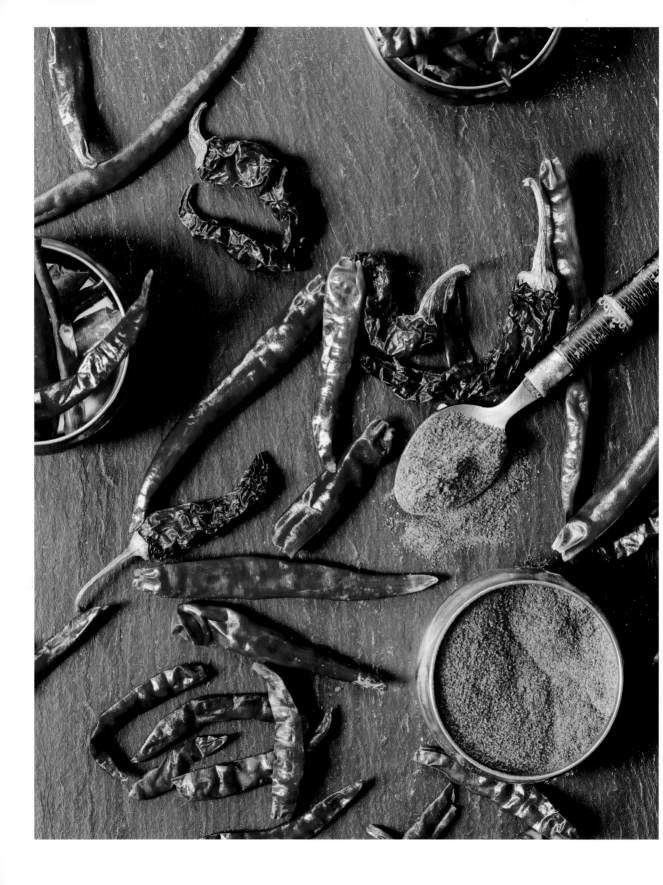

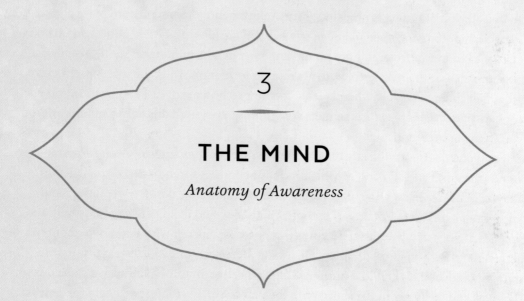

# THE MIND

*Anatomy of Awareness*

It would be easy to assume that the mind and the brain are the same thing. Technically, the brain is a fatty, jelly-like organ inside the skull that weighs about three pounds. It is responsible for motor functions like balance, autonomic functions like breathing, interpretation of the information brought in by the sense organs, and storage (memory).

However, Ayurveda sees the mind as separate from the brain. The mind is composed predominantly of subtle energies—even though you can't see them, they're there all the same. Mind is responsible for the movement of attention. For example, when you look at an object, your attention is pixilated; your attention moves from place to place all around the object, putting together an image of what you are looking at. The mind sees one point at a time but moves from point to point *very quickly*. The mind takes in the visual of the object, such as its texture or color, to get more information. Then the mind might make a judgment about the object, whether it's something to be liked or disliked, or the mind may compare it to other objects in the memory. All this happens in less than a minute without you trying or even noticing.

If you practice observing any object, you are practicing *awareness*. Awareness transcends the mind and can observe the mind's functions. Awareness can recognize the activity of the sense organs and thoughts, notice feelings like desire or repulsion, and know itself as separate from these thoughts, activities, and feelings. The philosophy and practice of yoga involve getting to know this observer, the self who is aware of thoughts and feelings. Because most of us exist in a state of mental confusion, we identify with thoughts and feelings and lose our sense of perspective. In this misinformed state, our thoughts and feelings run the show. With the practice of awareness, we begin to identify with our true consciousness (atman). In this state, we can achieve a sense of calm and peace, despite the continued, compelling presence of our thoughts and feelings.

## THE ANATOMY OF THE MIND

Some philosophies state that, because it can sense both the body and consciousness itself, the mind is a bridge between the body and ultimate consciousness, or the soul. The mind experiences, comprehends, and feels. Like the five senses, it is an organ of cognition. If you dissect a brain looking for the mind, you will not find it. Unlike the physical organ of the brain, the mind is composed of subtle energy rather than the five elements. If you studied an ear looking for the sense of hearing, it would be impossible; looking at the hardware of the ear does not let you put your finger on the energy that allows the ear to know a sound frequency, to hear.

The anatomy of the mind lies in its different frequencies, or functions. The higher mind comprehends eternal knowledge and universal truths about existence, the middle mind understands sensory experience and emotions, and the lower mind grasps only the physical world. Think of how you experience this range of functions—from inward and subtle, such as creativity and spirituality, to outward and earthbound, such as making a to-do list or remembering to pick up some milk. While Western models of the mind relate predominantly to thoughts, emotions, and memories, Vedic philosophy breaks down the mind into four parts that have different frequencies and functions. These functions are thought, comprehension, sensory awareness, and identity. Beyond the mind—linked to it but not limited by it—is the soul, or pure awareness.

You can cultivate higher frequencies through your food, your activities (such as meditation or selfless service), and where and with whom you hang out. Energy and matter operate on parallel planes that influence each other. For example, think of the energy you cultivate by eating fast food and watching a violent movie versus cooking a healthy meal at home and reading something inspirational. Our activities create different frequencies in us, and we are influenced by the frequencies of our food and surroundings.

## THE FIVE ELEMENTS AND THE FUNCTIONS OF MIND

Substances we ingest, the five elements, and their inherent energies are such an accessible way to work toward balance. To bring a tangible element to the subtle functions of the mind and the soul, we will match each of these frequencies to one of the five elements with a few examples of its qualities and energies. Space provides the undisturbed field where mind exists, while air is responsible for mind's movement. Fire is for discrimination, water for feeling, and earth for stability. These symbolic connections are merely to help you understand how the mind works and start thinking about the different ways remedies, food, and lifestyle can affect the mind.

### Atman and the Space Element

Atman, or pure consciousness, is not really part of the mind; it is *beyond* the mind—the space in which the mind moves, a formless awareness. It is our most universal, expansive aspect, and it is the least likely to be associated with the body or the constant fluctuations of thoughts and feelings. Atman illuminates the mind, like a lightbulb under a lampshade. We might consider this deepest layer to be our true nature that Ayurveda seeks to reveal. Remember, it is incredibly common to forget this aspect of ourselves, and forgetting is a root cause of disease. When we don't care for and identify with the pure aspects of our consciousness, life loses its spirit, and the deeper meanings of our existence are overshadowed by the day-to-day.

Space corresponds to atman and is light, dry, and expansive. The following are signs of the space element at work in the mind:

* Creativity inspired by having space for new ideas to manifest
* Spiritual focus and connection
* Spacing out, loss of focus and memory (too much space)

Substances that have similar qualities to atman and space include light, bitter tastes such as dandelion and lavender, as well as *prasad* (food as a devotional offering). A routine of waking before sunrise also cultivates a connection to atman.

## Citta and the Air Element

*Citta* is conditioned consciousness in which the spaciousness of atman contains personal experiences, memories, and thoughts. As you identify increasingly with your thoughts, the space of atman narrows. Think of citta as your personal field, a set acreage for this lifetime that you will plant and tend. Your thoughts and experiences are sown in the conscious, unconscious, and subconscious layers of this field. This means thoughts and experiences, whether you are aware of them or not, become part of your mind. The movies you watch, the remedies you take, the people you hang out with—all of them plant seeds in your field of individual consciousness. Maintaining tranquility in this layer of the mind is key to staying connected to the soul.

Air corresponds to citta and is mobile, light, and dry. Signs of the air element at work in the mind include:

* An active mind
* Being open to new ideas
* Sensitivity, becoming easily ruffled
* Racing thoughts and light, interrupted sleep (too much air)

Substances that have similar qualities to citta and air element are light and dry, such as coriander, turmeric, peppermint, and saffron. Stabilizing activities such as meditation and relaxation regulate the mobility of citta, as does following a consistent daily routine.

## Buddhi and the Fire Element

This sharp, focused aspect is the refined intelligence that is responsible for the mind's ability to discriminate, or know the difference between one thing and another. Buddhi digests and assimilates raw information, integrates concepts, and makes decisions. It bridges the inner and outer mental worlds through digestion and transformation. Buddhi makes judgments based on the information gained through experience and stored in citta. A luminous buddhi can shine on experiences to assess them truthfully, sifting through unorganized thoughts so as to generate intelligent insight.

Fire corresponds to buddhi and is intense, oily, hot, sharp, and penetrating. Here are some signs of the fire element at work in the mind:

- The ability to focus for long periods of time
- Efficient digestion and absorption of experiences and emotions
- Ambition
- A tendency to overdo things, impatience, obsessive thoughts (too much fire)

Substances that have similar qualities to buddhi and agni are hot and sharp and keep the mind alert, such as black pepper, chili, mustard seeds, and rosemary. Morning *dinacharya*, or daily routine, specifically cleansing of the sense organs, keeps the mind clear and fresh to perceive the world.

## Manas and the Water Element

This slightly sticky aspect of the mind flows outward through the five senses, gathering and absorbing information and sensation. It delivers raw information to buddhi. The word *manas* is sometimes used to mean all layers of the mind, but for now, we will think of manas as the mind that is concerned with sensory feeling—the mind with which most of us are familiar. The word *feeling* implies not only sensation but also subtle emotion. Manas relies on the outward-oriented function of the five sense organs: the ears, skin, eyes, tongue, and nose. It is through these organs that we receive information and impulses to act. Managing the outward movement of manas helps to maintain tranquility.

Water corresponds to manas and is slow, cool, smooth, and soft. Signs of the water element at work in the mind are:

- Empathy
- Attention to the external world
- A strong connection to the senses, especially taste

- Emotional intelligence, softness, and receptivity
- Being stuck in a rut, difficulty disengaging from ideas and/or people, moodiness (too much water element)

Substances with similar qualities to manas and water are soft, cooling, and moist, such as shatavari, milk, ghee, and anything prepared with love. Again, morning dinacharya to keep the sense organs free and clear keeps manas connecting to the world with fewer clouds and less confusion. *Abhyanga* (oil massage) is a wonderful way to support the skin's permeability to sensation and stimulation by keeping it supple and strong.

### Ahamkara and the Earth Element

Although ahamkara identifies with all five elements, it most closely corresponds to earth. The Sanskrit word literally means "I-maker" and is responsible for self-identification, or knowing that you are different from other people. The ego compiles the information from which self-identity results, and it tends to identify with only physical and mental processes ("I am a mother, a surgeon, a banker," and so on) rather than universal, spiritual processes. The most earthbound aspect of mind, ego is dense, stable, and resistant to change. It is from this level of mind that likes and dislikes, greed and self-interest, arise. Whereas our true nature is expansive, ego has tunnel vision and can lead to isolation. Ego is, however, a starting point for the process of all physical and mental functions from our first breath. Without the conscious evolution of mind, ego steals the show. It takes a lot of practice to learn how to observe the voice of the I-maker.

Earth corresponds to ahamkara and is slow, dense, stable, and heavy. Signs of earth element at work in the mind include:

- Strong memory
- Stability, resiliency
- Attachment, slow understanding of new concepts, resistance to change/new ideas, habit of living in the past (too much earth element)

Substances that have similar qualities to ahamkara and earth are heavy, dense, and stable, such as dates soaked in ghee (see the recipe for Jar o' Ojas on page 215), oil, eggplant, and meat. A tendency to overidentify with ahamkara can be kept in balance by practicing self-care with the larger goal of swastha in mind. This state of health pertains not only to the physical body but also to the mind and soul.

The Charaka Samhita tells us that it is wise to avoid mental agitations.[1] Mental imbalances are considered a huge factor in the disease process. The manovahasrotas, or channel of the mind, permeates the entire body. Think about how it feels when you get a sudden scare, like a close call when driving. Your whole body responds to an impulse sent by the brain. Doesn't it feel like the shock is present in every fiber of your being? It's a system-wide experience.

We could think of the mind as the control center behind the activity of daily life, like the Wizard of Oz. All the hubbub of Oz is being fabricated and controlled by a little person behind a screen. We go through life observing the illusions of the physical world as though this is all there is. When we pull aside the veil that clouds the mind, the inner workings are revealed. The journey of understanding the mind and, as often as possible, being aware of its processes leads to the ability to govern how we perceive and react to the world. If you bring your attention to perceiving your body in a healthful way, that vision of health permeates your entire body. While it inevitably takes more than mind power to heal and stay healthy, the attention and energy of the mind does have undeniable effects. The power of the mind to affect the body is due to what Ayurveda calls the subtle body, or energy body.

## PRACTICE TIP

While a healthy ego makes you strong and creative, in a state of imbalance, the voice of the I-maker can be like a broken record. If you pay attention to the stories it tells you about who and how you are, you may find that you keep listening to the same track; for example, *I am awesome, I am awful, I'm right, I'm wrong, I'm in control.* By applying awareness to the voice of ahamkara and knowing that you also have universal, spiritual aspects, these statements can begin to fall a little flat and eventually have less of a hold over you. This takes a long time and often requires an experienced guide—working with a counselor or meditation teacher can be a good place to start.

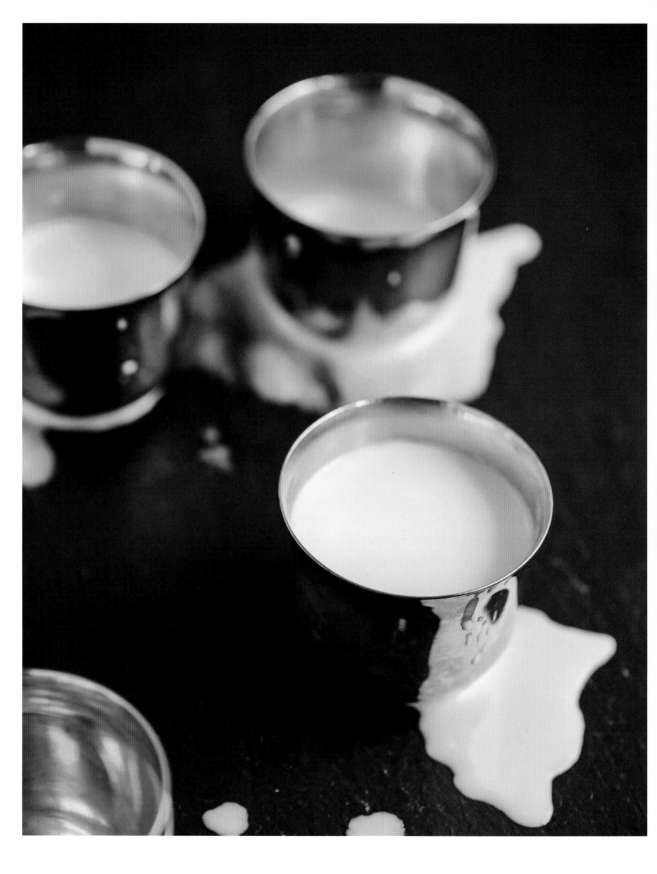

# 4

## THE SUBTLE BODY

*Vital Energy, Metabolic Transformation,*
*and Immunity*

That which can't be seen is *subtle*, while the physical world is *gross*. The subtle body is composed primarily of space, air, and fire elements. The gross body predominates in water and earth. The science of the subtle body is the specialty of yoga but an important part of Ayurvedic anatomy as well. As understood by the Ayurvedic definition of health, the subtle body cannot be separated from the physical body. The elements and tissues, the dhatus, and the doshas, in some respects, are physical, but without the subtle processes going on within, the physical body is dead.

The subtle body is made up of the mind and prana. It contains different levels of awareness, such as ego and intuition, and specific movements of prana, such as enlivening the senses and the movements responsible for vital processes. The yogic sciences describe the nadi system in detail, mapping the pathways that carry energy throughout the body. This information is not easy to come by, and it is intended to be experiential. The nadi system has some physical counterparts in the nervous system, but it is not limited to this physicality alone. The manovahasrotas is part of the nadi system. The mind travels in subtle channels, and it is through this system that the mind permeates and affects the body by influencing the way energy moves. Certain aspects of mind and energy are important in Ayurvedic practice, namely the subtle aspects of the doshas: prana, tejas, and ojas. Preservation of these three vital essences of the body is the heart of longevity.

## PRANA (LIFE ENERGY)

Prana is the energy of life. Because, like air, it is characterized by movement, prana is considered the subtle counterpart of vata. They work in tandem. This energy circulates around the body, carried by the currents of vata and governed by the movements of your attention. In cases of vata imbalance, the circulation of life energy can be compromised. For optimal health, prana and its smooth circulation must be cultivated with care. Moderate exercise, high-quality food, enough rest, good company, and self-love all build life energy. Mental afflictions, such as stress and worry, may be the biggest drain on life energy. A break in prana's rhythmic circulation can be physical, such as cholesterol blocking an artery or gas stuck in the intestines. However, psychic causes—chronic stress, worry, grief, or a general disconnect from the physical body (all computer, no exercise)—may be as important as physical causes in the modern progression of diseases.

### Prana and the Senses

An important part of the subtle body, the five senses are a major player in stress, important enough to earn them a ranking as one of the three causal factors of disease, trividha karana.

Eyeballs and earlobes may seem physical, but without prana, they are inert, and this, along with their intimate connection to mind, is why they are considered part of the subtle body. The survival instinct of the senses to be on alert to protect us and our young from dangers such as tigers and forest fires carries over into the present day. Survival instincts now are addressing ever more subtle causes, like financial strain and kids finding their way in the world. This persistent pull of the mental attention outward by the senses causes constant stimulation of the nervous system. If this natural outward movement of energy is not balanced by quiet time, heightened levels of stimulation result in stress and energy deficiency. Daily self-care practices address this phenomenon and preserve prana by nourishing and protecting the senses. A healthy daily regimen will result in less stress and more energy.

As we saw in pranavahasrotas, the channel of prana that begins at the nostrils and ends at the heart, this energy has a close relationship to respiration. Breathing is a life-giving activity and not to be ignored. Bringing the attention to the breath, at the heart of many yoga and meditation techniques, quiets the senses and the mind and nourishes the heart, the seat of prana. Rhythmic breathing is considered a vata-balancing therapy, and it can be as simple as the following breathing practice.

## SAMA VRTTI UJAAYI (EQUAL BREATHING PRACTICE)

*Sama* means "balanced," *vrtti* means "fluctuation," and *ujaayi* means "victorious." This breathing exercise makes one victorious over the fluctuations of the mind. It is accomplished by equalizing the fluctuations in the breath.

1. Sit comfortably, where you won't be disturbed, and set a timer for 5 minutes.
2. Close your eyes and take three breaths, just to settle in.
3. Begin to inhale and count from one to four as you go, landing on the end of the inhalation at four.
4. Begin to exhale and count slowly from one to four, completely emptying the breath at four.

Continue like this, counting rhythmically to four on each in- and out-breath. Concentrate on making them the same length and strength. This may take some practice. You may find that inhaling is easy and exhaling is hard, or vice versa. The counting is there to help you keep the rhythm. Stick with it, pay attention, and keep going until the timer goes off. Over time, you can increase your practice time incrementally, if you like. The more minutes you spend breathing in rhythm, the more stable and relaxed you will feel and the longer that feeling will stay with you.

## Full Prana Equals Full Power

In busy day-to-day life, it is very easy to lose touch with the movements of life energy and attention. A slow and steady commitment to paying attention to self-care and self-love pays off in the prana bank. Ayurveda excels at providing rejuvenating routines for all seasons and stages of life. Part two is full of them. Prana is the mainline to feeling full power and can bypass the physical body altogether.

## TEJAS

When you are on your self-care game and friends tell you you're "glowing," it's tejas at work. Think of tejas as the smoldering embers of fire that continue to emanate a gentle and sustainable source of energy once the fire has settled down. Tejas is the subtle aspect of balanced pitta dosha that governs the metabolism of food and information, and provides luster, luminosity, and brilliance to both body and intellect. Tejas brings a shiny glow to the skin, a sparkle to the eyes, and a sharp, clear mind. Tejas is responsible for a clear perception of the world around us, called sattva. In a balanced state, it burns through delusion and mental fog to reveal the true self.

Tejas is promoted by the intake of clean-burning fuel (nutritious food prepared with love), maintenance of a strong digestive fire, and the necessary time and space for the mind to process experience and emotion. Too much intake, the wrong kind of intake, or lack of energy and attention for transformation all compromise the body's luster. This is why retreats result in the glow; adequate rest and time for self-care and reflection are at the forefront of any retreat. A steady commitment to daily routine keeps the embers burning bright by keeping us in the habit of paying attention to wellness and carving out time to do what it takes to process daily living in the moment rather than playing catch-up all the time. Too much too fast, like wood on a fire, will overwhelm tejas, leading to a cloudy complexion and perception.

## OJAS

Unlike prana and tejas, ojas is a substance. Like cream as the essence of milk, ojas is the end product of digestion, produced once all the dhatus are nourished, and is the stuff of vitality and immunity. Charaka Samhita calls ojas "the nutrient cream of the body" and "that which keeps all the living beings refreshed."[1] Like honey, ojas is the nectar of nutrition, and it takes volumes of food and days of digesting to produce a small amount.

During the process of digestion and metabolism, a small amount of ojas is released into each tissue layer before the remaining nutrition is passed on to the next layer. This provides immunity and strength for each tissue. The refined end product, which takes thirty days to produce from food, results in ojas for the vitality and longevity of the entire body.

Burning ojas by overdoing it on a regular basis, or by subsisting on poorly digested food or not enough building food, shortens the life span. It takes one month of rejuvenation to make up for burning the candle at both ends. Keep in mind, you have to live large for a while to burn it up completely. Getting enough rest and rejuvenation time regularly is the way to promote strong immunity and true vigor. When you start to feel a decline in natural energy, take a rest to preserve ojas rather than pushing ahead all the time.

Ojas, tejas, and prana exist in a mutually beneficial relationship that sustains long-term health; their preservation is a fountain of youth. Healthy prana and tejas yield ojas from high-quality nutrition. Paying attention to healthy diet and routines and having a keen awareness of energy levels in both your body and your mind will result in high ojas.

### OJAS MILK

Dates, almonds, and cow's milk are prized substances because they contain a mixture of qualities that ultimately provide nutrition to build ojas (as long as they are digested well). These foods are commonly blended into a warm smoothie of sorts, called ojas milk. You will find variations on ojas milk with the addition of strengthening herbs and digestive spices in the rejuvenating tonic recipes in part three.

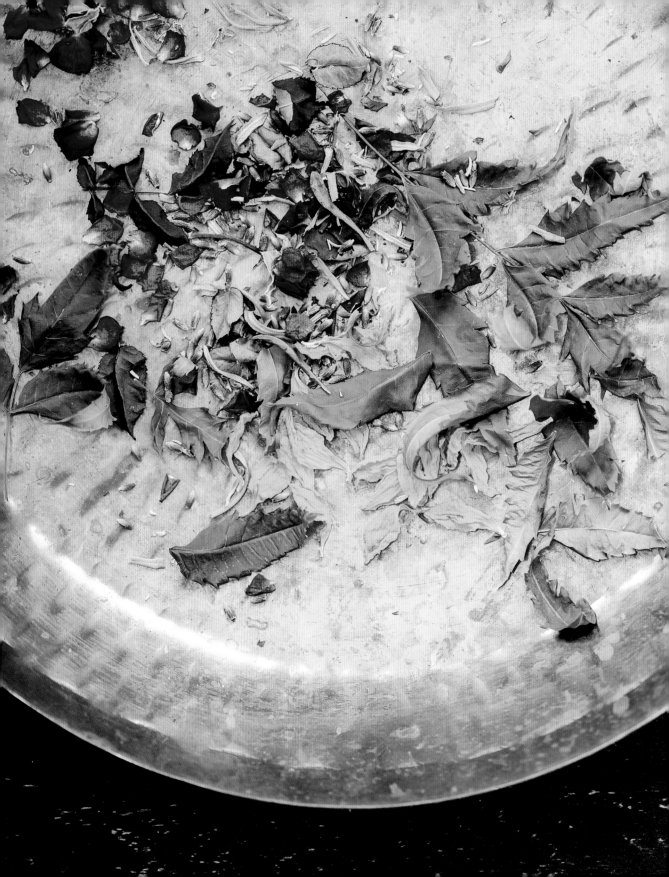

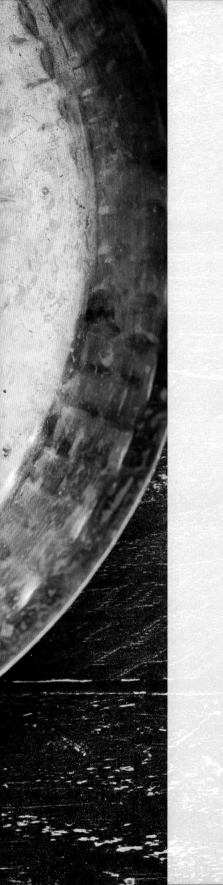

PART TWO

## *The* AYURVEDIC LIFESTYLE

—

DAILY AND
SEASONAL ROUTINES
FOR SELF-CARE

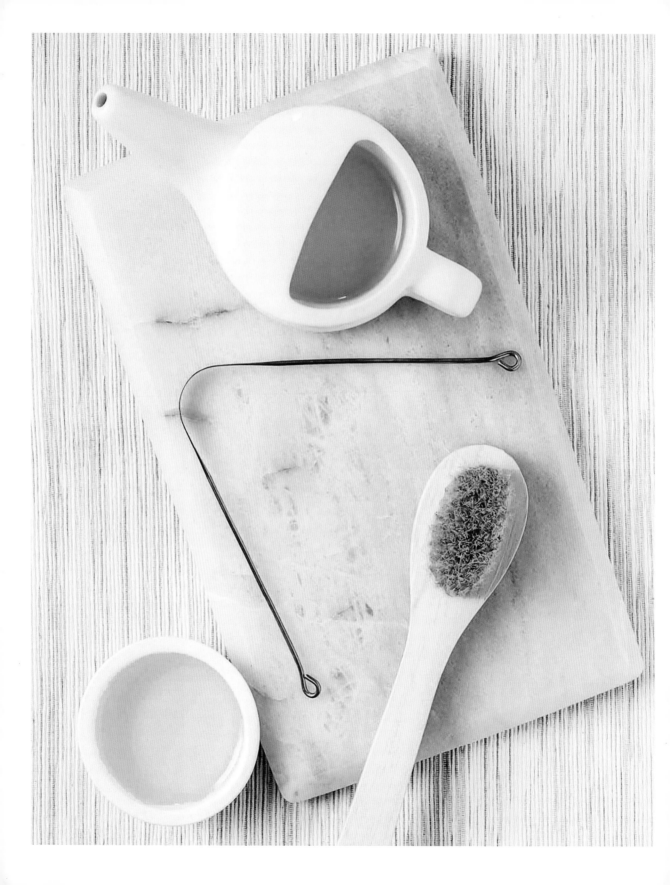

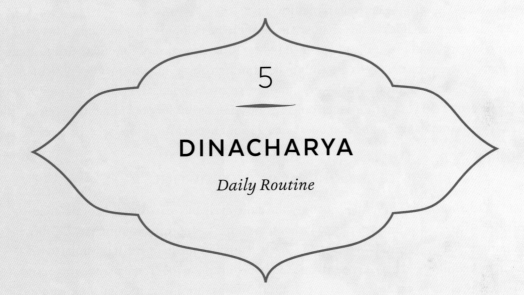

# 5

---

# DINACHARYA

*Daily Routine*

Dinacharya is an absolutely fundamental aspect of the Ayurvedic lifestyle for maintaining good health. The word means "daily routine." Due to the rhythms of nature, such as sunrise and sunset, certain changes in the body can be expected, like getting sleepy and hungry or waking up. The way the day naturally progresses affects the body and guides our days to move in unison with the cycle and to live in tandem with the natural energy sources that feed us. Waking, eating, exercising, and sleeping at the ideal time make everything smoother, and you will feel your energy become more buoyant as you move along with the currents of nature.

The general guidelines in this chapter are meant to be tailored to the individual needs of your body; for example, some people need to eat three times a day, for others twice a day is plenty. These personal needs are illuminated through observing the qualities present in your body. Understanding why these routines are recommended, and which qualities they promote, will help you decide which ones are most important for you, rather than blindly following a strict daily routine that does not take your needs into account.

## CLEANSING MORNING ROUTINES

The word *dinacharya* describes not only the daily cycle but also the body of practices performed at specific times of day to promote health. The morning routines are the most important, and here's why. While the body sleeps, detoxification happens. It is natural to wake up in the morning and have to pee, right? And hopefully poop too. There may be some crust in the eyes, perhaps a stale taste in the mouth. The doshas are always moving things around, transforming and digesting, building up the body, and these metabolic processes create waste, much as car exhaust results from running the car. On a regular basis, you change the fluids, clean the filters and hoses, and so on. Why should the body be different? This machine runs on food, and there are innumerable tubes in the body, the system of srotamsi, through which things are always moving. The channels that remove waste are the most important.

The tubes that open to the outside are two in the lower part of the body (the urethra and anus); seven in the head (two eyes, two ears, two nostrils, and a mouth); and the channels of sweat, which are innumerable, opening onto the skin. Thus, the morning cleansing routines of dinacharya involve pee, poop, care of the sense organs (eyes, ears, nose, mouth, skin), and exercise. These practices ensure that the tubes function at top form by keeping the openings of the tubes clear, so they don't back up and/or begin to accumulate gunk. Imagine a garden hose with sediment stuck on the end, just a trickle coming out, pressure building, hose swelling. I think you see my point!

Let's begin our day at sunrise.

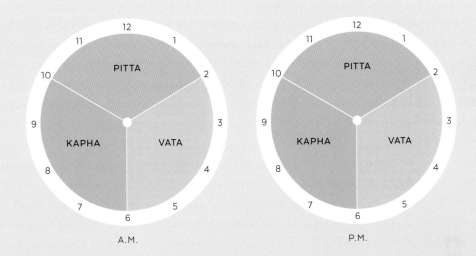

A.M.       P.M.

Due to changes in the sun, and its effect on moisture in the atmosphere, each dosha is more active at certain times of day. Knowledge of the pattern the doshas follow in a daily cycle will help in understanding dinacharya routines. For example, vata is most prevalent in the early morning, so many routines for the management of vata will happen during this cycle. The same is true for pitta at midday and kapha in the evening.

VATA is dominant in the early morning, between 2 A.M. and 6 A.M., and in the afternoon, from 2 P.M. to 6 P.M.

PITTA is dominant in the middle of the night, from 10 P.M. to 2 A.M., and in the middle of the day, from 10 A.M. to 2 P.M.

KAPHA is dominant in the late morning, between 6 A.M. and 10 A.M., and in early evening, from 6 P.M. to 10 P.M.

Here are a few ways the dosha cycles affect us throughout the day. Vata's light, clear, and mobile qualities make for a crisp wake-up with a clear mind before 6 A.M., but if vata is aggravated, it can promote feelings of being overwhelmed or tired in the afternoon cycle. A bit of rest in the afternoon will remedy this.

Pitta's sharp, hot, penetrating qualities make for a great time to digest a main meal at midday and an ideal time for "cooking" toxins out of the body in the middle of the night. Eating late will compromise this natural detox.

Kapha's heavy, dense, moist qualities make for a sluggish wake-up after 6 A.M. but a great time for exercise. The early evening is not the ideal time for a big meal when heavy qualities predominate, unless of course heavy qualities are needed.

## Wake-Up Time

It is recommended that you wake up before the sun rises. For those who are able to get to bed on the earlier side or don't need as much sleep, this time, known as *brahmamuhurta*, or "God's hour," is when both the external and the internal environments are most serene. Brahmamuhurta is roughly between 4 A.M. and 6 A.M. This time is good for studying, as the mind is undisturbed and the memory is strong, and for spiritual practice, contemplation, and meditation. The bodily wastes should be ripe for removal after sleep and clear easily during this time.

The 6 A.M. juncture marks the beginning of kapha time, and you can expect an increase in moisture in the body. In cases of dry constitution, this is a good thing, but this excess moisture builds in the body and can make waste products, such as mucus and poop, stickier, denser, and harder to remove. For those with a heavy, dense constitution, waking up after 6 A.M. will result in slower, more sluggish qualities in both body and mind. This unpleasant beginning to the day can be avoided by waking closer to, or even before, six o'clock. Give it a try and see for yourself: rise early for a few days in a row or even a week. You will notice a difference.

Note for northerners: During the time of year when the sun rises later, adjust your morning routine to be a bit later, perhaps an hour. It is natural to sleep more and rise a little later during the dark months.

It is very important to remember, however, that the recommendation to wake up between 4 A.M. and 6 A.M. applies only to those who wake feeling well-rested and enjoy complete digestion of their evening meal. This means one will have to poop soon upon waking. In order to savor the serenity of this special morning time, one must enjoy earlier evening mealtimes and an earlier bedtime. Generally, it doesn't have to be *all the time*. If you feel like giving this a try, adjust your evening and morning routines slowly and consistently, in increments as small as 15 minutes weekly. And it's OK if you get off track—new habits are not always easy. Give it some time.

## Cleansing the Channels

As already stated, the channels of elimination will be ripe for clearing upon waking (unless it's too early or late for you). Here are a few things to be sure to do.

ANSWER THE CALL. Go pee right away and poop if the urge is there. Do not check your phone first! If this is hard for you, turn off notifications or buy an old-school alarm clock so you are not tempted to engage with the screen immediately. Avoid multiple snoozings, especially if it means you will have to hurry upon waking.

**WASH YOUR EYES.** Run cool water from the tap and rinse your eyes well by keeping them open as you splash the cool water over them with your hands four or five times. Follow by blinking several times and rolling your eyes in circles.

**CLEAN YOUR MOUTH.** Traditionally, the gums and teeth would be rubbed with twigs of bitter shrubs, like neem. These days, go for toothbrushing and tongue scraping. Use a stainless steel or copper scraper, not a toothbrush, which will not clear mucus from your tongue. Before consuming any drinks, scrape your tongue five to six times, from as far back as you can get to the tip. Cover the entire surface of the tongue, especially way in the back. Press gently, but do not disturb the tongue tissue. Mucus will likely appear on the scraper; rinse in the sink as needed. After finishing, clean the scraper thoroughly with hot water, wipe dry, and keep it near your toothbrush. Do not scrape your tongue at other times of the day.

**GANDUSH (OIL PULLING).** The swishing or holding of oil in the mouth for 5-20 minutes is used to detoxify the cavities of the head and the digestive system, as well as to balance the effects of excessive air and space elements in the region of the head (this can present as vertigo, a spacey feeling, or pain in the jaw, ears, or scalp). As the minutes go by, the oil pulls saliva into the mouth, which cleanses the mouth of bacteria that can be responsible for tooth decay and bad breath. With longer durations, detoxification of the sinuses can also result in a small amount of drainage. The amount of liquid in the mouth will increase as the saliva arrives, and the oil should be white when you spit it out. As a preventive measure for oral hygiene and strong teeth and gums, practice gandush daily. If you don't make it happen every day, it still benefits you.

If you have a sensitive or dry mouth, use warm sesame oil. If you have sores or heat or itching in the mouth, use melted coconut oil or ghee. If you have excessive mucus or moisture, use warm salty water or triphala (see chapter 10) infusion.

Here's how to do it: Fill your mouth halfway with the liquid. In cases of vertigo or sensitivity of the head, ears, or eyes, allow the oil to sit in the mouth until saliva fills the cavity, then spit it out and rinse with warm water. In other cases, swish the oil for 5–20 minutes, then spit it out and rinse. Spit the oil into the trash rather than down the drain, as it can clog if you do this daily.

DRINK SOMETHING HOT. Follow gandush by drinking a few ounces of moderately hot water. Imagine the hot water melting and cleansing mucus from your head, mouth, throat, and stomach. If you have sluggish digestion, adding the juice of a quarter of a lemon to the water can help wake things up. I find that many coffee drinkers are really looking for a morning ritual as much as the substance itself. Lemon ginger tea can be quite satisfying.

TAKE IT SLOW. If you haven't had the urge to poop yet, it could be because you are running around the house getting ready or thinking about everything you have to do. It is very important to leave time and space for elimination, ideally before food. Consider 5–10 minutes of simply observing your breath or doing a breathing practice such as Equal Breathing (page 71). If that feels like a stretch right now, perhaps try a bit of inspirational reading or relaxed bird-watching out the window. Avoid reading the news if it gets you all worked up. Leave that for a little later. The idea here is to allow your mind to expand rather than narrow down to the small stuff. This may take practice, so hang in there.

## Abhyanga (Oil Massage)

The application of oil to the body is a longevity practice that nourishes and increases the resiliency of the body and nervous system. The texts say that those who practice oil massage are less susceptible to diseases and resistant to exhaustion and overexertion. Not to mention that regular oil massage is said to slow the aging process.[1] Such is the esteem in which this dinacharya practice is held. *Abhyanga* means specific movements applied to the limbs. The practice involves applying oil to the skin, head, ears, and feet and leaving it on for a while to digest before showering.

Massage is most effective for detoxifying the skin in the morning. However, oil's stabilizing qualities can also induce good sleep, pain relief, and relaxation when used in the evening. A coconut oil massage can cool the body in hot weather or calm inflammation. Because the skin needs to digest the oil, it is not recommended after eating or when ama is present. Oil's heavy, dense, moist qualities can increase ama.

### Amadea Morningstar's Turmeric Saltwater Gargle

When I asked Amadea, the renowned author of *Ayurvedic Cooking for Westerners*, what her top home remedy was, she offered this recipe. She says, "You can do a neti rinse if you like first thing in the morning, followed by this gargle. It's a great way to clear out excess kapha accumulated in the night."

**6 oz water**

**½ tsp ground turmeric**

**½ tsp pink salt**

Boil the water and pour it into a stainless steel or glass cup. Stir in the turmeric and salt. Cool to body temperature, then gargle for at least 1 minute.

## WHY NOT TRY A COFFEE SUBSTITUTE?

The heating, drying effects of coffee can be an instigator in pitta and vata imbalances. This recipe from *Everyday Ayurveda Cooking for a Calm, Clear Mind* is the coffee substitute I have seen work most often for clients—even in cases where a person was adamant about not giving up coffee. You can also use whatever sweetener or milk you are used to. If you can't kick the coffee, at least add cardamom to balance the acidity.

### Dandy-Latte

**2 cups water**

**1 tsp ground cardamom**

**2 tsp coconut sugar**

**¼ cup full-fat coconut milk**

**1 tbsp dandelion coffee powder
   (such as Dandy Blend)**

In a medium saucepan, bring the water, cardamom, coconut sugar, and coconut milk to a boil. Turn off the heat and leave the pot on the burner.

Add the coffee powder and foam the drink by using an electric milk foamer, whizzing with a hand blender for 1 minute, or mixing in a blender. Begin blending on low so the heat does not blow the lid off the blender; increase speed to high for 1 minute.

How you do self-massage is as important as when or what kind of oil you use. Some believe that simply applying the oil is the purpose, while others believe the massage itself is equally important. I would say to pay close attention to your vibe. Make sure you are not rushing, approaching this activity as just another pain-in-the-butt thing you have to do. Consider what a treat it is to have this time to care for yourself, and imagine all the benefits you are promoting for your body and mind with this ancient practice. Intend for self-massage to be an act of love. Foster gratitude for all of the functions the body is carrying out seam-lessly all the time, without any conscious effort. Reflect on how your attention pays off in the longevity bank, every and any time you perform an act of self-care.

HOW TO DO SELF-MASSAGE. Warm ¼ cup oil in a jar or bottle placed in hot water. I like to use a squeeze-top travel bottle, which is plastic, won't break, and makes the oil easy to dispense. Make sure the room you oil in is cozy and warm. Use a space heater if necessary. Prepare the room and remove your clothes before you begin, to minimize the need to go grab something (and the possibility of slicking surfaces with oil) once you start. Lay an old bath towel on the floor and sit down, or stand near the toilet or the side of the tub so you have a place to prop up a foot as needed. Breathe deeply a few times and give thanks for the time and space to care for yourself in this way.

First put a tablespoon of oil in your palm and apply it to the crown of your head (see page 84 for more about head massage). If you are not planning to wash your hair, do not oil your head. Use your palms to make wide circles over your face; avoid getting oil in your eyes. Oil your ears and the area behind them, using your little fingers to put oil in your ears and nose. Rub oil into the sides of your neck and across the tops of your shoulders.

Place a few tablespoons of oil in your palms and coat your arms and legs with it, getting more oil as necessary. Once your limbs are coated, vigorously rub the oil into your arms with long, downward strokes, then your legs. Use circular movements to massage your joints, and don't forget your fingers and toes. Apply more oil to your chest, abdomen, low back, and sides with large, clockwise, circular movements. Be gentle on your abdomen. Women should massage the breasts well. Use an up-and-down action on your breastbone.

Finish by massaging your feet well, using side-to-side strokes across the soles. I like to interlace my fingers between my toes and circle my ankles. When you've massaged in all the oil, lie back on your towel or in a moderately hot bath (this works well if your bath-room is chilly), and relax for 5–30 minutes. The massage should take about 10 minutes, and aim for at least another 10 minutes of rest. If you have to get going, even 5 minutes of massage, then a shower, is still beneficial. When you have more time, like on a weekend, let the oil soak in longer. The longer it soaks, the more benefits you will receive.

Now enjoy a hot shower, but wipe your feet first so you don't slip. Be careful! If there is any doubt about moving around when the feet are slippery, or any history of balance issues, skip the soles of the feet. Keep a little oil by your bed and do the feet at bedtime instead. Use a natural soap of lavender, sandalwood, or neem; the hot water will help remove the oil. Apply shampoo to the hair before wetting it, to cut the oil. After you shower, pat yourself dry. Your skin may still seem slightly oily, but it will gradually be absorbed. Afterward, clean your bathtub or shower stall of residual oil to make sure no one slips. I do this by spraying a little cleaner and rubbing it around with my feet. Baking soda, left for a few minutes, then wiped clean, will also absorb oil from the tub.

*Note:* When your towel becomes very oily, it can create a fire hazard if you put it in the dryer after washing. It's better to hang your abhyanga towels to dry and replace them periodically instead.

HOW OFTEN TO DO IT. As I said, anytime you practice is money in the health bank. Once a week is a minimum requirement. How frequently you need to oil depends on how dry your body is, stress levels, season, and age. Vata imbalance, pre- and postnatal, and frayed nerves are all important cases for frequent, if not daily, oil massage. If you notice more dry skin in winter, increase frequency to several days weekly; the same applies to periods of increased workload or stress and difficulty sleeping. As you get used to the practice, you will notice its effects and become aware of when an oil massage is needed. Soon enough, you will know what factors in your life increase dryness, mobility, and stress, and this will become a tool to balance those factors.

WHEN TO DO OIL MASSAGE
- In the morning for detoxification
- In the evening to improve sleep and quiet the nerves and sense organs
- After travel
- Anytime you need localized pain relief

WHEN NOT TO DO OIL MASSAGE
- After a meal
- When there is ama or indigestion
- During heavy days of the menstrual cycle
- When there is kapha aggravation or excess mucus
- In hot, humid weather

### QUICKIE MASSAGE

The texts say that oiling the ears and feet is most important. In the event you aren't making a self-massage happen very often, keep oil by your bed and massage a tablespoon into the crown of your head and the soles of your feet nightly. Depending on the type of hair you have, you may find you have to wash your hair in the morning or it will look a bit oiled. Wear a light pair of socks to bed to protect your sheets. Bonus: castor oil softens heavily calloused feet!

**WHAT KIND OF OIL TO USE.** Never use raw oils; use refined, whether you prepare them yourself or buy refined oils. This ensures that impurities have been removed, and you will notice refined oils do not have a strong smell. You may enjoy changing your massage oil with the seasons as indicated in the seasonal lifestyle guidelines, but here are a few general choices. Be sure to do a patch test with any oil before applying it to the entire body, to be sure you are not allergic.

- **Sesame oil:** Traditionally sesame oil is favored for its ability to build strength and softness in the body. Sesame oil is warming and indicated for those who run cold and experience dry skin.

- **Sunflower and almond oil:** These two lighter oils are neither heating nor cooling and are indicated for those who do not experience very dry skin, or those who don't absorb sesame well. These can be mixed with sesame oil.

- **Mustard oil:** Mustard oil is light and heating and stimulating for cool, heavy body types. This can be mixed with sunflower oil to find a comfortable amount of warmth.

- **Coconut oil:** Coconut oil is cooling and indicated for those who run hot or have sensitive skin.

- **Herbal massage oils:** A *thailam* is a base oil—commonly sesame, coconut, or sunflower—that has been cooked along with an herbal decoction to make a "medicated oil." You will find recipes for making herbal massage oils at home in chapter 10.

*Note:* Oils can also be blended together to achieve the ideal viscosity for your skin and season.

## Shiro Abhyanga (Head Massage)

This technique is excellent for relaxation and stress relief. Ayurvedic body treatments for the mind generally focus on the head, mouth, ears, and nasal passages for their proximity to the brain and the activity of the sense organs. Head massage and oiling of the ears and nose, as part of a full-body massage or alone, can be used to calm the mind. Because oiling the scalp must be followed by a good shampooing, practice the head massage weekly, when it is convenient for you to wash your hair afterward, such as on a weekend morning. When you have time, practice head massage to begin a full-body massage. When sleep is a problem, head massage can be an excellent way to calm the mind at bedtime. To avoid going to bed with a wet head, wrap your hair in an old towel, scarf, or hat and wash out the oil in the morning. Take care not to let your head get cold in the night. Head massage with oil is contraindicated in cases of congestion, fever, cold, flu, brain fog, and lethargy.

The oil used for the head is usually of a cooling potency and is applied at room temperature. Activity in the head region creates a lot of heat on its own, as I'm sure you've noticed! Coconut oil is cooling, or you may want to use sesame oil medicated with a cooling herb like *amalaki* or brahmi. Check out my Amalaki Triphala Hair Oil recipe on page 88.

If needed, heat the oil in a small vessel or ramekin. If you run cold, choose almond or sesame oil. Warm the oil slightly if it is cold out. Remove any hair ties and brush the tangles from your hair. Begin by gently kneading your shoulders and neck with circular motions a few times. Dip your fingers into the oil and distribute it evenly over your fingertips. Spread your fingers and work your hands into your hair on either side of your head, above your ears, with the fingers facing up. With a shampooing-like action, work your fingertips into the crown of your head. Rub the scalp around the crown of your head gently with oiled fingertips until you have covered the top of your head. This is the most important part of the scalp. Dip your fingers into the oil again and work the rest of your scalp until finished; this should take 5 minutes or more. Rub a bit of the oil onto the entire surface of each ear with small circular motions, and slide your pinky tips into the ear holes to coat them with oil. Wrap your head if it's bedtime, or relax for 10–30 minutes with the oil on your head, then wash it out.

To clean your hair, first apply shampoo to dry hair and work it into the first two inches or so from the roots. Add a small bit of water to make suds and shampoo. Add more water as needed to get enough suds for your whole head. Those with thick or porous hair may need to shampoo again to remove the oil. Sesame oil requires a bit more shampooing than coconut oil.

## Amalaki Triphala Hair Oil

*MAKES 16 OUNCES*  Using an herbal oil for massaging the scalp has benefits not only for the hair but also for the head, eyes, and ears. The oil can affect the quality and quantity of hair by stimulating the scalp. It is used to remedy hair loss, premature graying, and dandruff and to improve the overall strength of the hair. Used for head massage, this oil can be helpful in treating stress headaches, relaxing stiffness of the jaw and neck, and improving the strength and resiliency of the eyes and ears.

⅓ cup amalaki powder

⅓ cup triphala powder

2 qts water

16 oz unrefined coconut oil

### MAKE THE DECOCTION

In a wide saucepan over medium-low heat, combine the amalaki and triphala powders and water and boil the mixture slowly, uncovered, until the water is reduced to one quarter (16 oz). Do not use high heat, as it can burn the herbs. This may take 1–2 hours. Strain the amalaki and triphala out using a triple layer of cheesecloth inside a large metal strainer to hold the shape. Discard the herbs.

### INFUSE THE OIL

In a large, wide pan over low heat, add the oil and decoction and bring to a boil. Simmer until all the water has evaporated. You will be able to see and hear (like popcorn) the water bubbles disappearing. When it is finished, there will be no water bubbles and no popping sounds. Stir to be sure. This may take 2 hours.

Allow the oil to cool completely and transfer to a sterile glass jar with a tight lid.

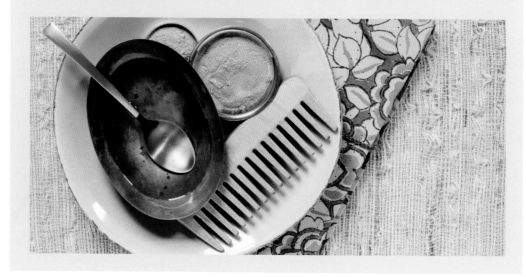

## Dry Brushing

This procedure is useful in cases of excessive moisture in the body and heavy, dense qualities, which can bring on lethargy, weight gain, or water retention. Dry brushing stimulates the body and mind and increases circulation. For those with heavy, moist kapha constitutions, it's a better choice than oiling, which can compound these qualities. Traditionally a practice called *udvartana* was used to remove moisture from the body by rubbing the entire body vigorously with a drying paste made of chickpea or mung bean flour. This is very messy to do at home, but an Ayurvedic bodyworker may be able to perform this for you. Gloves made of raw silk, called *garshana* gloves, can be used as a gentler option, where available. When you oil massage regularly, it is a good idea to do a gentle dry exfoliation to clear dead skin beforehand, once a week or so.

Use a natural-bristle dry brush (available in drugstores and health food stores) on dry skin. In a pinch, a rough washcloth will do. Beginning at the ankles and moving up toward the heart, make small, brisk circles to exfoliate and stimulate the skin of the entire body, especially the armpits and chest, inner thighs and groins, and anywhere stubborn fat tissue likes to hang around. Take 3–5 minutes and be firm, but do not disturb the skin. Emphasize the upstroke. A rosy color should result. Practice anywhere from daily to once a week, before your shower.

## Bathing

Bathing (or showering) in the morning is considered essential for good health. Imagine the innumerable pores on the skin being cleared out after a night's routine detox. Clarity of skin is also connected to clarity of mind and sense organs. What's not to love?

Hot water is best on the body for its ability to soften, melt, and remove wastes. The scalp and eyes, however, due to their tendency to accumulate heat, are best with warm or even cool water, depending on your climate. I am in the habit of a cool rinse of the head and back of the neck, even in colder weather. Since learning about Ayurveda, I have reduced the temperature of my shower a little bit. The skin should not appear red afterward. Hot showers can be drying for those with dry tendency; oil massage before bathing protects the skin, and one emerges with a soft and lubricated body. Use natural, moisturizing herbal soaps and shampoos and avoid fragrance and artificial cleansers. There are lots of natural Ayurvedic products, fancy as well as affordable, for skin and hair. Find some recommendations in the Resources section and recipes for homemade ones in part three.

# CARE OF THE EYES, NOSE, AND EARS

A little TLC for the organs that work hard for you all day every day is an important measure in preserving their optimal function. The senses are how you connect to the world around you, and keeping them clear, bright, and balanced will serve you well. This subcategory of dinacharya is best practiced in the morning so your senses are clear for the day, but it can also be used as needed when your eyes, ears, or nasal passages are under duress. If you have any history of imbalance or medical intervention with any of these organs, be sure to consult your doctor before practicing.

### Rose Water for the Eyes

If you have burning, itchy, or red eyes, you can spray or drop rose water into your eyes as part of your morning routine and any time of day that you need it. Be sure to purchase a hydrosol rather than water with essential oil added to it. Essential oils are not safe for the eyes. Hydrosols are made by steaming the plant in a closed vessel and collecting the water. Ayurvedic medicated eye drops may contain rose water, triphala, honey, castor oil, even onion, depending on the desired result. Conditions such as sties, burning eyes, and glaucoma are commonly treated with medicated drops.

*Note:* Do not put rose water in your eyes while wearing contact lenses.

### Nasya

Nasya is the administering of herbal medicines through the nasal cavity. These medicines may be for care of the sinuses, but just as likely for care of the brain and mind. Modern anatomy shows that nose-to-brain drugs can actually bypass the blood-brain barrier and reach the brain more easily. There are many nasya formulas for a variety of ailments, including strong treatments, which are administered only at panchakarma clinics.

There are two types of nasya: one is palliative, and one is cleansing. An oil infused with heating and drying herbs can clear up chronic congestion, while a palliative application of oil to dry nasal passages can calm the mind and provide a defense against bacteria and viruses. The air element is always moving in these passages, and lubrication is important for maintenance of health. A common formula for daily use is called *anu thailam* and is cleansing as well as lubricating. Plain sesame oil will keep the passages lubricated and protected.

Be sure that the oil and dropper that you use for nasya are absolutely sterile. I prefer to buy fresh nasya as needed in a two-ounce bottle from a trusted supplier (see Resources), just to be sure. Nasya can be done daily, as part of abhyanga in the morning and at other times of day as well. In very dry weather, I keep it by my bed and put a drop in my nostrils as needed before I go to sleep. Absolutely use it before you get on a plane!

1. Heat the oil by standing the dropper in warm water.
2. Tip your head back. (Or just lie down.)
3. Put two drops in each nostril, take a few deep breaths, and allow the oil to seep through. When you feel it has coated the passages, get up and spit out any mucus.
4. Rinse your mouth and gargle with a bit of warm water.

## Neti

Rinsing the nasal passages with warm salt water is beneficial for the prevention of mucus buildup and the removal of environmental pollutants, bacteria, and other bugs. In the event of increased moisture in the environment or in the sinuses, do not practice neti. The air indoors is often very dry when the heating or air conditioning is on, however, and if many of your hours are spent indoors, the damp weather may not be what you are working with.

I see people who swear that by doing neti every day, their allergies and general sniffly nature are a thing of the past. These are often kapha types. For others, neti doesn't drain well and can cause a bogged-down feeling in the head; it may possibly even compound sinus issues. A general way to approach nasal irrigation is as a cleanser, when needed. For example, after a dusty, dirty ride, after being around an allergen or sick people, after a plane ride—in all these cases a nasal wash can rinse out something unwelcome and possibly prevent a cold. I am religious about a neti after flying, when the heaters come on in the fall, and during the cold and flu season, for maybe two weeks.

In the event of excessive mucus, do not do neti. Inhalation of a stimulating, drying substance such as eucalyptus would be better. Traditionally, inhalation of herbal smoke was used during the rainy season.

HOW TO DO NETI

1. Boil purified water and add enough cold purified water to be sure it is not too hot. You should be able to hold your finger in it without burning yourself. Be sure to check.
2. Dissolve fine-grain, pure sea salt completely in the warm water. (Neti pots come in different sizes, so read the instructions on yours to find the correct amount of salt.)
3. In the shower or at the sink, lean forward, keeping the back of your neck extended so your whole torso is bent. Tip your head, place the spout into the top nostril, and wait for the water to run out the other nostril. If the water does not drain easily after a few tries, refrain from practicing until you can get formal guidance. Let the water run out naturally.

Do not forcibly blow your nose, as this can send the water in farther, which can affect your ear. You may cover one nostril and simply exhale to help the last bit of water out.

4. Tip your head the other way and repeat for the other nostril.

*Note:* Too much salt burns; too little leaves you feeling like you have swimmer's ear. Do not practice neti more than once a day or before lying down. If you have a history of sinus or ear problems, or are in any doubt about whether neti is good for you, consult your doctor.

### Karna Purana (Ear Oiling)

*Karna* means "ear," and oiling your ears can help reduce stiff neck and jaw, lessen ringing in the ears, and soften earwax. This is a vata balancing therapy that brings a feeling of calm and can induce sound sleep. It is especially useful as a weekly practice in cold weather.

What I notice for many people, vata types especially, is the way neck and jaw tension gums up the circulation around their ears and can eventually, in a subtle way, hinder the energy moving in the ears. After some time, this can affect the ears' ability to discharge earwax and cause changes in the resiliency of the delicate bones in the ears and actual hearing function. Now, this is a long-term process that started out with stress tension, which at some point might have been softened or tempered a little by some ear oiling. I'm a big fan, and a weekly dose is worth the few minutes it takes.

HOW TO DO KARNA PURANA

1. Use sesame oil for its antibacterial properties. Warm a glass tincture bottle of oil by standing it in hot water, or put a little oil in a cup and stand that in hot water.
2. Lie down and apply about five drops in one ear (if you're using oil in a cup, use a cotton ball to drop the oil into your ear). Close the ear flap with a finger and rub in circular motions for about thirty seconds. Next rub the entire ear, your jaw, and behind the ear for about one minute.
3. Put a cotton ball in the ear and turn over to repeat for the other ear. Keep the cotton balls in for a half hour or so; if it's bedtime, sleep with them in your ears.

Ears are a big deal and connect to the throat and the sinus, so if you have any doubt about whether ear oiling is safe for you, or if you have consistent ear pain or discharge, talk to your doctor.

## Garlic Ear Oil

**MAKES 2 TABLESPOONS** Oiling the ears can be used in cold, dry weather to prevent earaches and impaction of earwax. It can also relieve ear and jaw pain. I swear by it when I feel like I'm getting a cold. Garlic oil is used in many cultures for its antibacterial properties to treat earache and infection. It is extremely heating and "cooks" out bugs, as well as makes the ears, nose, and throat region inhospitable to bacteria and viruses during the cold season. It is very easy to make and works best when fresh. Look for garlic cloves with purple streaks on the peel, as they will be the strongest.

**1 clove garlic**

**2 tbsp sesame or olive oil**

**1 glass tincture bottle**

Peel and crush the garlic clove.

In a small saucepan over low heat, warm the oil.

Once it is warm, not hot, add the garlic and swirl together until fragrant. Allow to cook for 5 more minutes on low.

Remove from the heat, pull out and discard the garlic, and pour the oil into the glass bottle. Let it cool enough to use. Store it in the tincture bottle and stand the bottle in hot water for 1–2 minutes before each use to warm the oil. Never put cold oil in your ears.

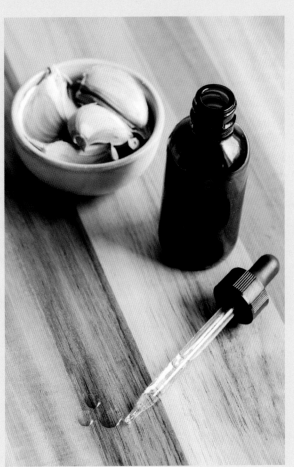

Exercise and diet are also an important part of a daily routine. The amount of exercise and food you need may vary at different times of the day, year, and stage of life. The right amount is unique to you. Let's look into the factors to consider about wise exercise and food choices.

### Exercise

Traditionally speaking, exercise is considered that which makes the body tired. It increases lightness of the body, brings endurance and the ability to withstand hard work, increases agni, reduces fat, and defines muscle tissue.[2] Those with heavier, denser builds, those who consume rich foods regularly, and those who live in cold climates should exercise to half capacity, while those in warmer climates and of lighter build should be even more moderate.

I find this to be quite different from the Western view of exercise. Exercise is thought of as something that brings energy rather than makes the body tired. Due to the often sedentary lifestyle of the developed world (watching TV, desk jobs where eight hours are spent sitting) and the availability of unlimited quantities of food, it makes sense that exercise feels energizing. Many bodies need it, really badly.

As with all things Ayurveda, the questions remain, for whom is exercise beneficial, and in what amount, at what time of day and year? How much is too much, and who should avoid it altogether? The more-is-better mentality applied to exercise can get you in a pickle. Understanding the right amount and how that amount may change at times can be a great tool for energy management in both body and mind.

General recommendations are that you should exercise until your breathing becomes fast, your mouth gets dry, or sweat begins to form on your forehead, nose, and spine. Then it's time to cool down. The idea is not to wring out your body but just to get the circulation moving, warm things up a bit, and call it good. A moderate daily routine for longevity might include walking, swimming, easy jogging, tai chi, or yoga. In the case of excess fat tissue, more exercise is OK, according to individual capacity. That's not to say if you are a lover of bodybuilding or marathon running that you are on the wrong track, but know that vigorous exercise, going beyond the half capacity recommended, is a hobby that needs to be balanced by adequate rest, recovery time (perhaps an oil massage), and nourishing diet. When we push too hard, the body can dry out, the dhatus undergo depletion, doshas become aggravated, and we burn up our ojas.

A lack of physical activity, however, can cause its own problems. An overload of unremoved wastes, clogged channels, or dense and slow qualities can begin to shroud the body—and soon, the mind as well. This is most likely in those with earth and water constitutions who can happily remove some moisture (mucus) by sweating and are likely to sweat more profusely once they get going. Exercise is the number-one management for kapha types. Coupled with a lighter diet, these folks enjoy the strongest body type that withstands all sorts of stressors.

The season is an important factor, because hot weather makes the body tired, whereas cold weather makes the body stronger but also harder and slower. Exercise is more important for warmth and circulation in winter and spring. The funny thing is, living in a cold city, I notice how many people stop exercising in winter, then dust off the sneakers and get back outside in warm weather. Exercise is key to managing a long winter and will make the heavy, damp spring season much lighter.

The right amount of exercise should feel refreshing, not tiring. The ideal of "fitness" in Ayurveda is not of muscle sculpting but of balancing the doshas, removing wastes, and getting the right amount of nourishment to the tissues.

### Ahara (Food)

One of the daily routines we all engage in is eating. Meals are not always considered an act of self-care, but here's where the message of Ayurveda is so important today. Food is our number-one substance for maintaining the health of the body and absolutely deserves our attention and care. If you've seen one of my cookbooks, you know this already, and those books are a great resource for learning more about balancing your unique body with food.

As part of a health-maintenance program, Ayurveda texts go into detail about *how* to eat as a separate topic from *what* to eat. The how takes into account certain factors that may change how efficiently food is digested, such as whether it is served hot or cold and the texture and quantity of the food. Most important, however, are eating habits. Habits are actions repeated regularly, often without our noticing. We continue to gravitate toward behavior that is familiar to us, unless we are paying close attention and trying to make a change. In this way, habits may be the most potent aspect of how we nourish ourselves (or gunk ourselves up) because they are happening all the time. Charaka Samhita defines healthy and unhealthy habits related to food as most important. Healthy habits are the ones that ensure good digestion, while unhealthy habits compromise the digestive process.

WHEN TO EAT. The time of day a food is ingested makes a huge difference in how it digests and metabolizes. Eating foods with the same qualities of the dosha most active at that time of day can increase the likelihood of imbalances. For example, ice cream aggravates kapha. It is cool, moist, oily, heavy, and dense. Kapha is most prevalent between 6 and 10, A.M. and P.M.

| HEALTHY EATING HABITS | UNHEALTHY EATING HABITS |
|---|---|
| • Eating after a shower (bathing increases agni) | • Showering after eating |
| • Eating when hungry (not suppressing hunger) | • Overeating or eating when you're not hungry |
| • Eating until you're two-thirds full | • Sleeping after eating |
| • Eating more than two hours before bedtime | • Exercising after eating |
| • Eating warm, moist, slightly oily foods | • Eating while distracted (working, talking too much, being on a smartphone, and so on) |
| • Eating your main meal at midday | • Skipping meals; grazing |
| • Sitting down to eat | • Drinking ice water with meals |

Eating ice cream during those times will create a load of these qualities. Imagine eating ice cream for breakfast when you wake up at 9 A.M. feeling groggy. Doesn't sound very balancing, does it? Many people are in the habit of eating ice cream at night, as a treat at the end of the day to ground the body, cool a stressed-out gut, or please the mind. Ice cream before bed is going to sit in the gut longer at night due to lack of movement and activity, as well as lack of sunlight, nature's agni. The heavy, dense, moist aspects of the cold cream will become thicker and stickier, harder to digest, and more likely to end up as fat, or ama. Ice cream at midday is more likely to digest and metabolize while you move around and the sun is at its zenith, warming the cosmos.

### KATE O'DONNELL EATS ICE CREAM

I'm from New England, the region of the United States that eats more ice cream than any other. I eat ice cream. For lunch. On an empty stomach. Followed by a big walk. No more food until I'm really hungry. And that is the only way I eat ice cream. I enjoy it—and I digest it.

Dry, cold foods are going to be most aggravating in the early morning and late afternoon vata cycles (beware the afternoon munching on chips and popcorn). Spicy, fried foods are going to be most aggravating late at night (midnight pizza fest). At midday, more foods are going to digest well, no matter their qualities. Be smart, and enjoy!

The thing to know about sleep is that there is an ideal time for it. Sleeping between the hours of 10 P.M. and 2 A.M. ensures the body's ability to harness the second cycle of pitta and use that heat and penetrating quality to cook out toxins. A lot of organ cleansing and regeneration happens during sleep—the nighttime kind. In the wee hours of the morning, the body pushes the toxins to the channels of elimination. The timing of sleeping and waking makes all the difference in supporting the body's ability to get rid of junk.

Around 6 P.M., kapha and its slow, heavy qualities begin to accumulate, increasing until 10 P.M. As that hour approaches, it is the ideal time to begin slowing down, disengaging from work and screen time, and preparing for sleep. Staying awake past 10 P.M. or 11 P.M. will compromise the body's detox time. Eating a heavy meal after 8 P.M. will increase the heavy quality, as well as require digestion during sleep, when agni in the stomach is low. Sleep and digestion do not go well together! Allowing for at least two hours between food and bed will ensure healthy digestion and sound sleep.

There's good sleep and bad sleep. Good sleep happens naturally at nighttime, between sunset and sunrise. Not-so-good sleep happens in the day and can be the result of exhaustion, disease, depression, or overeating. Sleeping in the daytime increases kapha, which may result in low agni, congestion, sluggishness, and weight gain. In cases of physical or mental exhaustion, sleeping during the day may be necessary for a time. Those with weak constitutions and the elderly may enjoy a healthy habit of daytime napping.

### NIGHT OWLS

According to Ayurveda, there are no "night owls" in the human realm. That is like classifying a "day owl" or a "day rat." Nature is nature, and human beings sleep at night. In the event of working night shifts, caring for a baby, and other unavoidable factors that hinder sleeping at night, you can maintain good health with a consistent schedule, including some self-care practices and rhythmic sleep cycles that follow a daily clock in accordance with your needs. The key is to be consistent.

**TOO LITTLE SLEEP.** Most people suffer from lack of sleep rather than an excess these days. Ayurveda texts define the causes and management of lack of sleep, which generally occurs in those with a vata imbalance, the elderly, and the overworked. In some cases it is an individual's nature to suffer from lack of sleep. There are many reasons people suffer from lack of sleep. These might include:

- Excessive cleansing
- Fear, anxiety, anger
- Uncomfortable bed or sleeping quarters
- Suppression of sleepiness
- Dry food (too much raw food, popcorn, crackers, and so on)
- Overwork
- Change in sleeping time (jet lag)
- Too much screen time

There are things you can do to help your insomnia or lack of sleep:

- Eat moist, grounding foods, such as milk, ghee, wheat, takra, soups and stews, and herbal teas.
- Drink ghee and milk (see Lubrication Station recipe, page 204).
- Try a head massage and/or foot massage with sesame oil or brahmi oil. Applying a small amount of oil to the crown of the head by making small circles on the scalp with the fingertips can improve sleep.
- Be sure the sleeping place is not too hot or cold and smells pleasant. Apply a dab of lavender oil on the temples.
- Think positive thoughts. Remember achievements, give thanks, visualize picturesque places.

In my experience, the most common problems affecting people's sleep are going all day without resting the senses, lack of a regular sleep routine, using screens at night, and suppression of tamas, the natural urge to slow down. It's OK to feel tired! If the day is very stimulating, expect that it will take some time to wind down. If you lie down in the bed and experience racing thoughts, these recommendations can likely help you sleep better. Eat a warm and easy-to-digest dinner, massage your feet with oil, and turn off the screens before 10 P.M.!

## SELF-CARE FOR HAPPINESS AND BEAUTY

Beauty is often mentioned in the Ayurvedic texts, through delicate seasonal beverages, aesthetic dishware, fresh flowers, adornments, and scented oils. While longevity is a science, it is also an art, and there's nothing wrong with enjoying and nourishing the natural beauty of the body when you have the time and resources. So many of these dinacharya routines can be approached in the way you might approach a mani-pedi or a newly tailored suit. Self-care can be a necessity and an indulgence, a delicious balance of attention paid to health, in a way that increases quality of life not only for yourself but for all those you come in contact with.

Daily routines are a big topic. There may be several changes to consider if your habits are far from this ideal or if you are not in the habit of paying attention to the time or your body. I notice when I teach this topic, people start to get a little overwhelmed. It's easy to focus on all the things you're doing wrong. It's also easy to think, *I'm going to do it all tomorrow!* Both of these attitudes can be hard to work with. In the first, one might think, *forget it then*. In the second, burnout is imminent.

Habits hinge on each other, as a daily routine winds along a path of interdependent activities. The time you get hungry for lunch depends on when you had breakfast. The time you fall asleep depends on the time you woke up that day. Adding or changing even one of these routines is significant. Go ahead, pick an easy one, and see how it changes you. I'll bet you come back for more.

And remember, bodies want to be healthy—it's their job. Helping them out a bit with wise choices is a great practice that adds up to a longer, happier life.

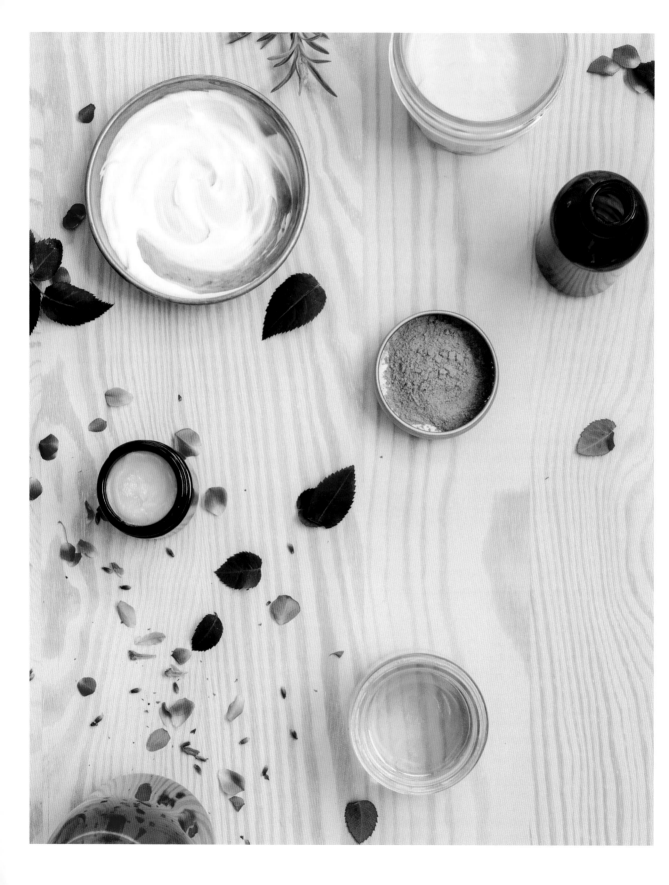

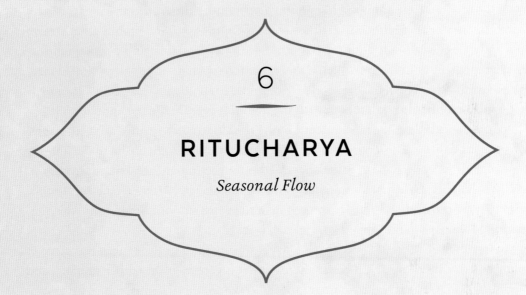

# 6

---

# RITUCHARYA

*Seasonal Flow*

*Ritu* means "season," and an understanding of the expected changes in the environment and how these affect us underlies the efficacy of seasonal routines. In the same way that doshas are more active at times of day that exhibit similar qualities to them, seasons can increase and decrease the doshas and their qualities. While the ancient texts discuss six seasons on the Indian subcontinent, these seasons are defined by the proximity of the Earth to the sun. In this way, any place on the planet will exhibit its own seasonal flow based on how that part of the planet is tilting toward or away from the sun.

Of the original six seasons, each spanning two months, three are warm and three are cool. Hot weather has reducing qualities—such as light, sharp, and mobile—that weaken the body. Cool weather is building in nature, with heavy, stable, and dense qualities that strengthen the body. Too much reducing or too much building causes imbalance, so essentially changes in the diet or daily routine are intended to maintain a balance of reducing and building, in tandem with the qualities present during annual cycles.

Ayurveda texts describe the tendency of the doshas to accumulate during a season of similar qualities. This accumulation holds the potential for a dosha to become aggravated—an early stage of imbalance. Without proper management, these seasonal changes hold the potential for impending dosha imbalances. *Ritucharya* is the science of pacifying the doshas as the seasons change to keep a smooth flow within, despite expected changes in the climate.

A temperate environment may have four seasons, while a tropical place may have two: rainy and dry. In the northern hemisphere, winter is generally December, January, and February, while these are the summer months in the southern hemisphere. Historically, people paid close attention to the seasons for agriculture, and many cultural festivals and annual calendars still revolve around the importance of local crops, although today farming practices may be the last thing on most people's minds. The knowledge of environmental changes and how they affect us is a bit of a lost art, but it is something that can benefit modern folks in very practical ways.

Rather than simply laying out a seasonal plan, which may not coincide with everyone's geography, let us investigate why certain routines are considered beneficial at certain times of year. Once you understand the qualities being managed, you can make the call based on what you experience in your home place. Every location changes throughout the year, and even small changes will feel big to those who are used to consistency. There will be certain factors about changing weather that are noticeable to everyone, and some helpful signs and symptoms about your health to keep an eye out for. For those who travel, keep in mind that the activity and frequent changes to your environment can aggravate vata, making it important to look to fall and winter routines to pacify vata during travel.

It's easy to superimpose this information on your climate, but time has its own program. While you might decide "spring" is March, April, and May, it might turn out a little differently from year to year. Knowledge of the world is subject to reality, so stay present!

## WINTER

Winter is described as that time when Earth is tilting away from the sun, making the environment colder and darker. Without the drying heat of bright sun, winter starts out with more moisture. There is precipitation, either as rain or snow. Something else to consider these days, however, is the climate indoors. If a place is cold enough to require heaters inside, this heat is going to dry out the air. If you spend a lot of time indoors in winter, dryness in the body will result, especially in the respiratory channels. This is important and may require more effort toward moisturizing practices such as oil massage and nasya. Dryness in general increases as freezing temperatures bind up moisture in the air.

Equally important is the way the digestive fire responds to the lack of sun. In cold weather, the fires of the body recede into the digestive organs. The fire in the stomach will be stronger, and the capacity to digest more and heavier food increases. In cold weather, foods with sour, sweet, and salty tastes are favored and better digested. These building tastes will feed the stronger fires, while a light diet in winter can set the body up for deficiency. It's easy to notice an increase in your appetite when the temperature drops, and it's natural to start baking seasonal favorites like pies and casseroles. Go for it!

If you have dry, light, cold qualities in the body, vata imbalances are more likely. This is the time of year to be on your oiling game. If you have a hot constitution, you will feel refreshed and stronger this time of year.

### Diet

- Favor sweet, sour, and salty tastes.
- Enjoy foods that build the body, such as wheat and oats, meat if you eat it, root vegetables, bananas, dates, and sugar cane.
- Enjoy a moderate amount of foods that warm the body, such as ferments, warming spices, cashews, pickles, citrus fruits, and olives.
- Enjoy foods that moisturize the body, such as sesame, dairy, almonds, ghee, and olive oil. If you don't get enough good fats, you may begin to notice dry stools or dry skin.

◆ This is the time of year for rejuvenating tonics (see chapter 10) that support the immune system and stave off deficiencies.

### Dinacharya

Sleep when the sun goes down, which means you get more sleep! It's natural to get tired earlier and stay in bed a little later this time of year.

Practice oil massage at least once a week with sesame oil. Follow with a hot bath. Practice neti as needed or use a nasya oil. Cover your head and ears when you go into the cold, and keep warm in general. Drink warm herbal waters such as ajwain, cumin, ginger, and cinnamon. Throat Soother Tea (see page 191) contains licorice, which increases moisture in the channels.

### Exercise

Since the body is stronger and slower in winter, up the exercise a bit. Daily movement will keep the tejas burning bright and circulate warmth as well as moisture throughout the body. Since you're eating heavier foods, you'll do well to keep your metabolism up. When you experience dryness in the body, however, be wary of too much sweating.

## SPRING

Spring is the damp time of year that follows winter. The earth will be full of new growth, and temperatures will be on the rise. In very cold places, spring is marked by the thaw, when freezing temperatures are finished for the year. This change from dry and cold to moist and warmer (or at least no longer freezing) causes a very particular reaction in the body. To balance winter dry and cold air, the moist quality of kapha has accumulated during winter, and as winter goes on, mucus can become thick in some places, like the lungs or sinuses. When the temperature rises, this mucus begins to melt and fill up spaces in the body. This may cause sinus and chest congestion, low agni, a tendency toward colds and allergies, and even lymphatic congestion. Ayurveda texts recommend certain measures to cleanse the body of this excessive moisture, but it is important not to practice them until winter is over. This could be as early as March and as late as May in the northern hemisphere.

Those who live in tropical climates may never have a winter but will likely experience a rainy season. The spring regimens are very helpful for managing an increase in moisture during the rains. This is a time when colds, congestion, and low agni are likely. If you have more moisture in the body to begin with, spring will be a heavy time when digestion slows down and your body feels thick, maybe a little water-logged. If you have a dry, light body type, you may feel grounded and rejuvenated at this time of year.

### Diet

* Favor pungent, bitter, and astringent tastes.
* Enjoy foods that warm the body, such as ferments, honey, spices, and lemon.
* Enjoy foods that dry and lighten the body, such as barley, corn, millet, legumes, prunes, berries, and greens.
* This is the time of year when a vegan diet can be beneficial.
* Avoid too much moist, heavy food, such as dairy, potatoes, fried foods, and sweets.
* Do not consume cold drinks or smoothies.
* Do not eat when you're not hungry.

Most of the medicines described in the ancient texts are liquids, herbal wines and waters that mobilize and cleanse the rasa dhatu. Drink warm herbal waters with a bitter, astringent taste, such as fenugreek, tulsi, turmeric, and *moringa*. Adding honey can help scrape thicker mucus from the body and adds warmth. Cumin-Coriander-Fennel Tea (page 183) is very helpful in keeping the agni strong if you suffer from a lack of appetite. There are a handful of kashayams and herbal honeys in chapter 10 for congestion and low agni. The rainier the weather, the more important all of these recipes and recommendations will be.

### Dinacharya

The cavities where moisture tends to accumulate are most important in spring: the throat, mouth, lungs, sinuses, and stomach. A strong nasya oil that contains astringent herbs can help keep the sinus cavities clear. Use oil in the nose only as a preventive measure and never when there is congestion. Saltwater gargles and oil pulling cleanse the mouth and throat. Oil massage will become less important, while dry brushing will invigorate and mobilize the blood. A dry sauna is an excellent way to remove some moisture from the lungs, sinuses, and entire body. Avoid sleeping in the daytime, which increases kapha, except in cases of illness or exhaustion.

### Exercise

Spring is the number-one time for exercise, which removes moisture through sweating, melts kapha by building heat, and mobilizes the lymphatic system that is responsible for flushing out winter accumulation. Exercise also builds agni and improves appetite. First thing in the morning is the best time, on an empty stomach, to remove excess kapha. Yoga to build up a light sweat, jogging, or cardio will do the trick. It is wise not to eat until you are hungry. On a heavy, rainy day, you may notice a lack of appetite, so eat less. Within an hour after exercise, it is likely your appetite will improve.

## SUMMER

Summer is hot! It may be dry and it may be humid, depending on location, but sunshine and heat will be present. The effect of the sun is to evaporate moisture, so in general, heat is drying to both the earth and the body (since sweating dehydrates). For those in coastal or tropical regions, there may also be a good deal of humidity. Imagine how you feel after getting too much sun, and you can understand how heat weakens the body. Promoting moisture and keeping cool is the key to avoiding imbalances of pitta dosha, which accumulates in hot weather. This can result in skin problems, acid indigestion, or feeling irritable, puffy, and overheated. These symptoms may not show up until the season is well under way, but they will continue to increase as the months go by.

During summer, agni circulates throughout the entire body and is less strong in the stomach than in winter. This brings a lighter appetite, when heavy, oily foods will compound heat and can block the channels. If you have more fire element in the body, you will feel tired out and quick to anger during summer. If you naturally run cold, you will feel more comfortable and energetic. Keep in mind that in very hot climates where life is lived in air conditioning, the air indoors will be very dry.

### Diet

- Favor sweet, bitter, and astringent tastes.
- Avoid things that heat the body from within, such as alcohol, ferments, spicy food, and acidic fruits and vegetables such as oranges and tomatoes.
- Enjoy lighter foods, such as legumes, rice, quinoa, coconut, juicy sweet fruits, and fresh cooling vegetables such as cucumber and zucchini.
- A plant-based diet works well in summer, when so many varieties are in season.

Many bitter and astringent-tasting spices can be enjoyed as cool herbal waters, especially fennel, coriander, mint, cardamom, and lavender. These drinks, taken regularly, will hydrate the body as well as cool the blood. If heat is getting blocked in your digestive tract (sometimes a reaction to dehydration from dry heat is constipation), have Triphala Tea (see page 184) at night until the heat feels relieved.

Ayurveda texts make special mention of rice, milk, sugar, grapes, and coconut water for their ability to cool the body. In this respect, grapes are considered the king of fruits (see Cardamom-Ginger Grape Elixir on page 253). Aloe vera is a very bitter plant that can be used to make juice that cools the body, which is why we have a section of aloe coolers in chapter 10. A thin rice kanjee, served at room temperature or even cool, is another healing food to hydrate and nourish when your appetite is low (see page 218). If you have a stronger appetite, you can make it with almond or cow's milk instead of water.

### Dinacharya

If you are in air conditioning, be sure your unit is clean. If your nostrils feel dry, practice nasya. Stay out of the midday sun and wear a wide-brimmed hat. The head reacts strongly to heat, so keep it cool and save yourself the headache. Finish showers with a thirty-second cool rinse, especially on your head and the back of your neck.

Because heat is expelled through the digestive tract and skin, it is important to keep these two channels clear. Overeating and consuming heating foods and alcohol will not make you feel well. Instead of eating a large midday meal, you may shift to a bigger breakfast before the day heats up and a moderate dinner after it cools down. In general, more fruits and vegetables and less dense, slow-to-digest foods will keep the digestive tract clear so heat can be removed, and symptoms like swelling and acid stomach will be less likely.

Avoid using antiperspirant or heavy creams and conventional body oils, which can block the pores that release heat. Eating less garlic and onion in hot weather will help keep the body cooler and the sweat less stinky. A coconut oil massage can remove heat from the body and protect against sun damage and dryness. Neem is among the most bitter and cooling of Ayurveda's herbs, and infused into coconut oil, it is ideal for a dry, hot climate (see recipe on page 250). In extreme humidity, oiling your body may be the last thing you want to do. Go with that feeling and have a cool bath or shower, and try aloe vera gel instead of oil.

In summer, preserve your strength and limit activities that increase heat, such as exercise classes in hot rooms, jogging under the sun, and vigorous cardio. Get in the habit of doing an exercise routine in the early morning, before the day heats up. Keep it cool with walks near water or in the woods, swimming, and slow yoga. Be sure to enjoy a cool, not iced, drink after exercise.

## FALL

The fall season is generally marked by cooler temperatures, increasing winds, and dryness. As summer shifts into cooler weather, the body will want to get rid of excess heat accumulated throughout the summer months. How the fall goes will be a function of how the summer was. If it was a hot one, and you indulged in heating foods and activities, you may experience a pitta imbalance. It is natural for the body to experience a mild increase in heat when it is hot out, and diet and lifestyle can calm or aggravate this heat during the season. Fall is an important time *not* to increase heat and oiliness, as pitta dosha may be mildly aggravated. If the winds are up in fall, they will blow on the heat, in the way one blows on a fire to get it going. This can cause flare-ups in the digestion, skin, and beyond. If you have a hot constitution, you will benefit most from this knowledge. If you run cold and dry, you may miss the summer qualities and need to do more to manage the drying effect of the rising wind and cool weather.

### Diet

- Favor bitter, sweet, and astringent tastes. Reduce foods that heat the inside of the body like chilies, fried foods, alcohol, raw onions, and garlic. Keep things simple to avoid sour food combinations, and do not eat until the previous meal has been digested. Even taking time off from snacking can be enough to allow digestion to clear out some heat. Eating lesser amounts of food in general will help the agni clear the channels.
- Enjoy foods that are easy to digest and enhance clear channels, such as mung beans, rice, ripe fruits, especially grapes and melons, and fresh vegetables, especially greens. Soups and stews are good. Watch out for clogging foods, such as yogurt, cheese, and fatty meats.
- Amalaki is a rejuvenating herb for pitta and will benefit all body types. Try taking 1 teaspoon daily with a bit of hot water for a month or so.

- Moringa is a cleansing herb to relieve accumulated heat. See Moringa Coconut Water recipe (page 170).
- If the appetite is good, Brahmi Ghee is a nourishing tonic that will be grounding for hot as well as dry types. Try taking 1 teaspoon daily with a bit of hot water before breakfast for a few days or one week.

### Dinacharya

If it's back-to-school time, practicing neti for a few weeks can help rinse away potential cold bugs. Dust is blown around once the heaters get turned on in cold climates, which also makes it a good idea to rinse the nasal passages. Once the season turns dry, provided there is no congestion or allergies, look to nasya for the cold weather.

Oil massage is a great fall practice to ground the body, balance rising dryness, and soften the channels so the body can expel heat. Choose an oil based on the qualities you are experiencing, and try to practice the massage a few times weekly. It can be excellent to do an oil massage daily for one week as the season changes.

### Exercise

Rest is in order to allow the body to recalibrate at this time of year. If your usual routine is vigorous, back off a little for a few weeks and do less than you are used to. Use the extra time for an oil massage. Avoid catching a chill by running in the cold; favor brisk walks, swimming, and moderate yoga to circulate energy and ground the body. Stay out of the wind or cover up.

## RITUSANDHI

The transition between seasons is a very important time in an Ayurvedic lifestyle. Texts describe a two-week period when the weather changes back and forth between the previous season and the one that is rising. During this time it is ideal to begin dropping the routines from the previous season and adopting the routines for the coming season. It makes sense that life doesn't change in a day, so routines need to shift gently over a few weeks. Gradual change is easier to adopt and easier for the body to adjust to. Too much too fast can itself be a cause of imbalances.

I am often asked how to know when the season is new—one day it's hot, the next day very cold, and people become confused. After a year or two of observing your environment, it will become easier to recognize this period of changing qualities. You might even notice that you naturally adopt different routines based on your cravings. For instance, fruit salad may not sound as appealing as oatmeal on a cold, blustery morning. That means it's time to grocery shop and begin to restock the pantry. Changes in temperature and moisture are good attention-getters. Watch for such signs as dry skin or scalp, cold hands and feet, loss of appetite or heavy stomach, and oily skin and hair. Think about how these signs can tell you that your body is becoming dry, moist, overheated, and so on.

Spring is the time to get rid of heavy, moist, dense, slow qualities that accumulated during the winter. The longer your winter is, the more important spring cleansing may be. Fall is the time to get rid of hot, sharp, penetrating qualities that accumulated during the summer. For hot body types, this can be very important.

A spring cleanse for the management of kapha dosha may include:

- More exercise, especially outdoors
- Sweating, via working out or a dry sauna
- Dry, light foods (served warm if it's still cold out)
- Neti and nasya to clear the nasal passages
- Dry brushing
- Triphala Tea (see page 184) or saltwater gargling

A fall cleanse for the management of pitta may include:

- Relaxation time—less moving around and more lying around
- Cooling foods served warm, with plenty of ghee
- Neti and nasya, if needed
- Sesame oil massage and/or coconut head massage
- Herbal waters

### What to Consider before You Cleanse

A seasonal cleanse can be a good way to shift seasons. Eating a simple diet and practicing daily oil massage help the body to clear out any aggravated dosha by increasing agni and clearing the channels of elimination. It is not a more-cleansing-is-better kind of thing, and there are many individual factors to consider about whether it's the right time to cleanse. Cleansing can also be a clearing of old habits, energy patterns, or messy desk space. The point is to slow down enough to take stock of your daily rhythms, your diet, and your dinacharya practices and see how they are serving you. Are some qualities in need of balance? Perhaps the oil you are using is too thick or too thin for the present qualities, perhaps the spices you usually cook with are too heating or cooling;

## SPRING CLEANSE FLOW

Try the following program for three to seven days when winter is turning into spring. Recognize when the air feels moist and temperatures are well above freezing.

- In the morning, scrape your tongue and gargle for 1–2 minutes with warm saltwater or Triphala Tea (see page 184).
- Exercise on an empty stomach.
- Dry brush, then do neti or nasya in the shower.
- Eat Mucus-Busting Kanjee (see page 217) and/or Spicy Dandelion Green Soup (see page 224) for at least one meal per day.
- Eat sit-down meals of warm grains, quinoa, buckwheat, amaranth, corn, and legumes that are light on fats and include plenty of cooked vegetables, especially those of bitter and astringent taste. Avoid sweets, potatoes, and dairy.
- Eat Ginger Blaster (see page 231) before meals, one to three times each day.
- Drink Cumin-Coriander-Fennel Tea (see page 183) throughout the day, or mix 1 teaspoon of Spicy Hot Honey (see page 198) into hot water.
- Drink warm Fenugreek Water (see page 169) or Tulsi Water (see page 173) often.
- At night, drink Triphala Tea and do nasya unless you are congested.

## FALL CLEANSE FLOW

Try the following program for three to seven days during the period of summer shifting into fall. Recognize the shift by the increasing dryness, cooler temperatures, and possible winds.

- In the morning, scrape your tongue and have 1 teaspoon of Brahmi Ghee (see page 239) in hot water.
- Take time for contemplation, meditation, or pranayama and a walk outdoors. Do not rush the morning.
- Do an oil massage for at least 20 minutes.
- Eat sit-down meals of kanjee for breakfast and whole-grain and vegetable soups and stews. Follow with After-Meal Chewing Spice Mix (see page 232).
- Avoid alcohol, coffee, and spicy foods.
- Drink 4 ounces of Homemade Aloe Juice (see page 176) after lunch or dinner.
- Drink Summertime Cumin-Coriander-Fennel Tea (see page 183) or Mint Water (see page 169) throughout the day.
- At night, drink Triphala Tea (see page 184) and oil the nose if your nasal passages feel dry.

maybe it's time for hot lunches instead of salads. It's best to keep a broad view of what cleansing means and to be in the moment as seasonal junctures arise so you can decide what is beneficial at that time.

The state of your agni and dhatus is important. Knowing when to introduce building qualities and when to introduce reducing ones makes all the difference. You must be strong enough to cleanse without creating a deficiency in any of your tissues. If you have zero body fat, you should not lose weight in the name of a seasonal health regimen. For you, undertaking a cleanse might look like not drinking coffee and eating junk food and eating only foods that nourish your body. This allows a cleanup of your system. But it also requires a focus on nourishment and the preparation of good food, possibly more than three times daily. Cooking, grocery shopping, and sitting down for meals are all important steps.

A big problem I see often is people wanting to take on a cleansing diet but keeping up the same rigorous lifestyle. This is a no-go. Rest is an essential aspect of Ayurvedic cleansing. If your attention and senses are going outward all day, your body requires nourishment—juice won't cut it. Your inner channels, which may indeed be in need of a sweep and mop, will not receive care from your body when your attention is focused outward most of the time.

Equally important is the body's need to rebuild after a cleansing period. This process of rejuvenation, known as *rasayana*, is an important part of a cleanse and a specialty of Ayurveda.

### Rasayana

Rasayana ("rus-AY-ahna"), the science of rejuvenation, is a jewel of Ayurveda. The word describes that which promotes longevity and prevents aging and disease. Rasayana can be achieved through lifestyle regimens, as described in chapter 5, as well as through diet and herbal medicines. You will recognize the word *rasa* from rasa dhatu, the first tissue layer—an unctuous layer that circulates through the entire body responsible for maintaining nutrition and immunity. Rasayana is the practice of creating excellence in rasa dhatu. This excellence will then translate into the nutrition of all the tissue layers and cells in the body. Don't forget that the quantity of rasa dhatu is only one part of excellence; its free circulation throughout the body is also key.

Foods that are sweet in taste and cool in potency, like sugar, milk, coconut, and ghee, are ideal for building rasa and are often found in rasayana formulas. These foods maintain the nutritive, liquid, and unctuous qualities of the dhatu. They are often paired with penetrating digestive spices to help these qualities reach the deep tissues, such as pepper, ginger, and cinnamon. Hot and dry reproductive tissue is not ideal, and this can

## CULTURAL CHANGES

Changes to the daily routine are not due to nature alone. Culture can also be a factor in lifestyle rhythms and have a huge impact on health. In some places, fall is a time of massive change in daily schedules as children and university students go back to school, and they as well as their families are swept into a sudden shift in the demands and timetable of daily life. It is wise to take into account the effects such changes have on the system. If you think about it, it makes sense that digestion, sleep, or nerves might go through the ringer a bit as things are suddenly quite busy and quite different from how they were a week or two before. Simplifying your diet and implementing a few touchstone routines, such as a consistent lunchtime or bedtime, can make things run a lot smoother while change is afoot.

Adopting a diet and routines that calm heat and allow the body to expel any excess is key this time of year. A consistent daily routine will balance the fluctuations experienced during stressful times. Consistency of routine may be the most important factor for maintaining health, especially in vata types who are unsettled by changes.

result from too much stress, depleted ojas, overexercising, or an excessively heating diet. People with more fire in their constitution will be more prone to the effects of heat. Heat will, over time, dry out tissues the way a candle left burning underneath a wood table will begin to dry out the wood. It takes a little time, but it is inevitable. Slowing down for self-care is an important part of remedying this trifecta of heat, dryness, and depletion.

Sometimes herbs or spices of heating potency are headliners in traditional rasayana formulas, such as ashwagandha rasayana, and these are ideal for cold weather, vata imbalance, or people of cold constitution. Knowing when to call on heat and when to call on cool is an important distinction among rasayana substances, as is a clear sense of what the agni can digest.

Ashtanga Hrdayam says that "rasayana given to someone who has not completed shodhana (cleansing) first is like trying to dye a dirty cloth."[1] This means the nutrition will not stick around. The tissues need to be prepared to receive it first. Substances such as herbal milk or ghee will be better received after a light diet, for example, when the body will absorb the fats and their medicines easily. Taking an herbal milk after a burger and fries might just overload the agni. So, it's helpful to think about rejuvenation as a practice that works in tandem with healthy digestive practices, and maybe even cleansing if necessary.

It's easy to get so busy that external changes go by without notice. That's why the ancient Ayurveda practice of observing seasonal changes can be such a great help today. Observation naturally illuminates the wisdom of living in relationship to nature. The aspects of life that are true and undeniable—change, age, hunger, thirst, sleeping, waking—speak to us as soon as we start listening. Through ritucharya we learn to listen and respond to the changes around us. The right thing to do at any given time becomes clear through presence as well as practice.

## A CASE STUDY

Nicole was a former triathlete who ran on the track team in high school and college. When I met her, she was twenty-six and experiencing instability in the joints and irregular periods. Years of overexerting the muscle layer had left her joints and uterus lacking in nutritive fluid. The muscle layer had been sucking up all the juice. The goal was to introduce the right kind of nutrition to rebuild these tissues, such as ghee, milk, and coconut oil. The problem, Nicole said, was that when she ate these foods, she felt heavy and sleepy after and wasn't able to keep up with her day.

Nicole had been eating a raw foods diet for about one year when we met, and her agni was unaccustomed to breaking down heavier, denser foods. First, we had to build up her agni and improve absorption with deepana and pachana spices added to her cooking, and a focus on relaxed, sit-down meals. After some time she began to feel comfortable digesting a little more food at mealtimes. We introduced a mixture of coconut milk and ghee at bedtime with warming spices, and she reported that she found it very grounding and delicious and felt she slept better after this tonic. With time, she started feeling more relaxed and restful in general, her desire for warm cooked foods increased, her tendency toward overexercising decreased, and she began to notice the correlation between a light diet and cracking and discomfort in her joints. Within six months, her periods became regular, provided she kept her exercise regimen moderate.

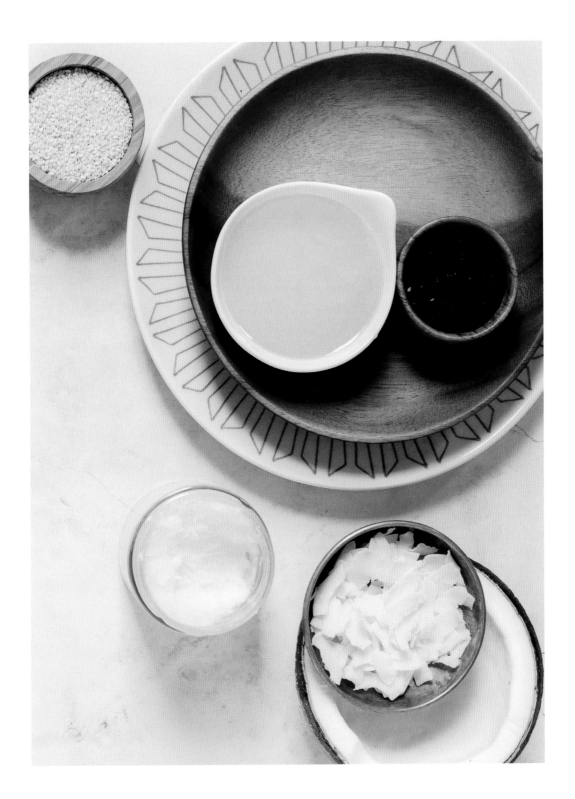

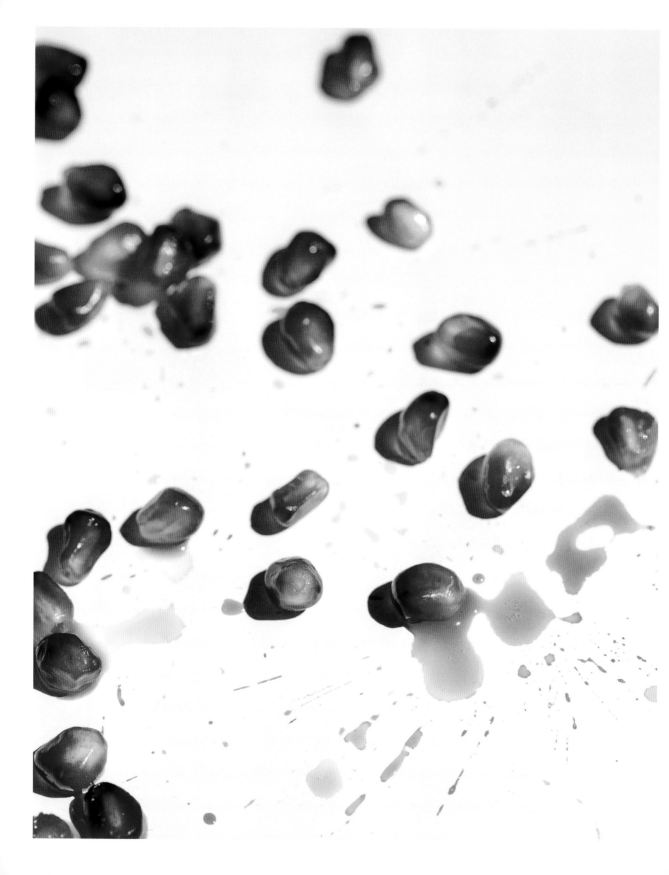

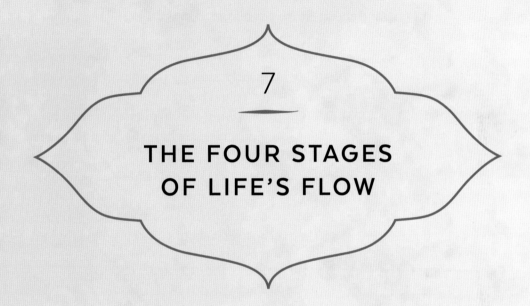

# 7

## THE FOUR STAGES
## OF LIFE'S FLOW

In the preservation of health, Ayurveda takes into account not only the time of day and time of year but also the time of life a person is in. Learning this concept in my late twenties revolutionized the way I thought about my life. Certain aspects, qualities, and even doshas are prevalent at different life stages. The Vedic view of life clearly describes four stages of evolution that dovetail with the four components of life: body, mind, senses, and soul. Life begins with a building of the physical body, then a sharpening of the intellect. The active years naturally give way to a slow reduction of stimulation, more peace and quiet. As we age, the time and energy we have to devote to spirituality and the life of the soul increases.

I find this life flow invaluable in understanding the bigger picture of the arc of my life and not getting stuck on the small stuff or mindlessly fostering imbalances. I spent a few long trips to India in my early twenties traveling around pretty aimlessly but quite sure that I *wasn't* going to buy into the cultural norms in my own country and get a job, get married, buy a house, have kids. Of course, I didn't have any life experience to give me a context for finding what I did want. I was lost.

An Indian activist in her early sixties suggested that I was doing life backward. She pointed to my dreadlocks and said, "You are living like a mendicant, but you haven't lived your life yet. You don't know what you are renouncing." She was very kind and very wise, and though I felt defensive, I had a feeling she was right about something. But I couldn't tell what. It was some years later, as I began to tire of the "freedom" that comes with a transient life, that I learned about the concept of the four *ashramas*, or stages of life, and those wise words began to make sense.

## BRAHMACHARYA

Do you remember, as a child, someone saying, "One cookie is enough" or "You're overtired. It's bedtime"? As kids, we don't really know that eating the whole box of cookies is going to cause problems or that we will go crazy if we don't get enough sleep. Certain things we learn are "not right," while others are. Learning about what is right and wrong for us as individuals, and as members of a community, is what *brahmacharya* is about. In the yoga system, these principles are called *yamas* and *niyamas*, personal and social observances such as nonviolence, cleanliness, and truthfulness.

Brahmacharya can be translated as *brahma*, the "divine," and *charya*, "movement"– moving in a way that is harmonious with the divine (much as dinacharya is moving in a way that is harmonious with daily rhythms). It doesn't have to be a religious thing; learning how to live in the world is a practical endeavor.

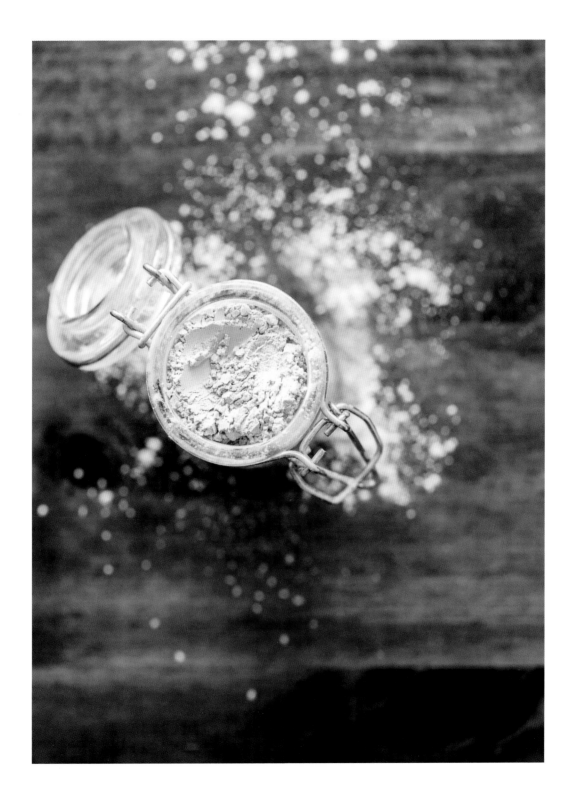

These first twenty-five years or so of life are a time of learning. It is important to support young people in gaining perspective on the world and how to find meaning in it. Brahmacharya is about the *how* of life, not the what. The development of a sound moral and spiritual compass, an understanding that life requires nourishment and attention both internally and externally, is the best-case scenario for these younger years. If during this stage of life we are taught that only material success matters, we are set up to work in that direction in the second stage of life and end up wondering what it's all about when that stage shifts.

Brahmacharya is the kapha time of life. The building qualities of kapha support the growing body, strengthen the immune system, and provide a pliant mind to collect experiences and memories.

## GRIHASTHA

I think of "householding" as taking care of the business of daily life. In this second stage of life (roughly age twenty-five to fifty) of *grihastha*, the focus is on engaging with the external world, being a part of a community or society, working, making money, having a family, acquiring stuff. You are no longer a child; you need to stand on your own and find security and sustenance—and perhaps even provide for others as well. This is a time of action and responsibility. The moral background learned in the first stage of life governs the activities of this second stage. Holding down the responsibilities of an employee, a partner, and/or a parent may easily take up most of your time. The pursuit of self-knowledge might fall by the wayside and is often not a priority. While these years are intensely busy for many, setting aside time for routines that keep you grounded and healthy will ease the transition into the next stage.

The activity of this stage will remind you of the hot, sharp, intense nature of pitta, and indeed this is the pitta time of life. An awareness of balancing pitta dosha with relaxation time, nature, and play—in addition to keeping stimulants (coffee!) and recreational drugs and alcohol under control—will help keep things in balance despite what may be a very busy time. This stage goes on for a few decades, so take a long view and pace yourself!

## VANAPRASTHA

In this stage of life, roughly from age fifty to seventy-five, half of life is behind you. The idea of "forest dwelling," or *vanaprastha*, is a retreat of sorts—taking a step back, not all the way into a cave, just retiring out of the city and into the quietude of forest living.

As the responsibilities of the active years wane, it is time to shift your attention toward the inner life more and more. This doesn't require moving or being in the actual forest (though that sure inspires contemplation), but it does require making space for a sense of self that is not dependent on job or family. It is at this time that it becomes clear, if you lost track there for a while, that you are not your responsibilities or your achievements, not your job, not just a parent, but a luminous heart!

This can be a hard time for those who aren't used to resting or dwelling on the deeper aspects of being alive. In a culture where productivity is often at the top of the ladder, a shift toward doing less can bring on a midlife crisis. I, for one, am so grateful for this aspect of my Ayurveda studies, which has helped me enrich my grihastha years with simple daily practices that keep me grounded in myself, while keeping an eye on my tendency to rely on outward success for meaning in life.

The shift into vanaprastha begins the vata time of life. For women, this corresponds with menopause; for men, there is a less marked transition but a shift all the same. The growth governed by kapha and the hormonal activity of pitta both recede, and the body becomes subtler. It is time to focus on managing the qualities of vata dosha—dry, cold, light, and so on—through Ayurveda's longevity techniques, such as oiling the skin and increasing oils in the diet.

## SANNYASA

The word *sannyasa* suggests a wandering ascetic. While wandering may not be in the cards for most of us, the final stage of life, at maybe seventy-five to a hundred years, is a time for withdrawal from the likes and dislikes, the doing and desiring, that have characterized life thus far. The idea is that beginning to disengage from the objects of this world before death will make dying a lot smoother. With a little preparation, we might go with a sense of satisfaction and find the prospect of death much less intimidating. This final stage of life is a time of connecting deeply to the spiritual aspects of life without much distraction. Now that's something to look forward to.

These stages of life are a guideline, not an absolute, and not everyone is going to experience life in this pattern. Maybe you started out backward, like me. Maybe a lot of it is already behind you, but it is never too early or too late to understand the framework of a life cycle and what this may reveal about living wisely *now*.

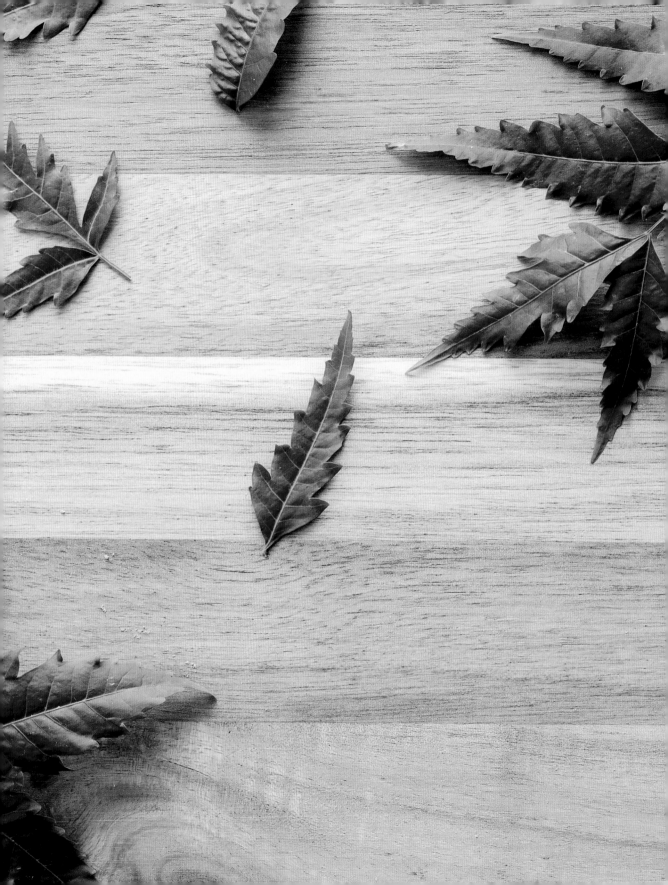

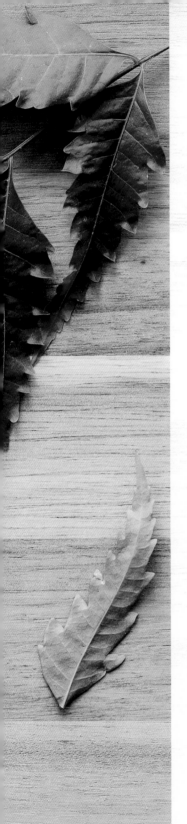
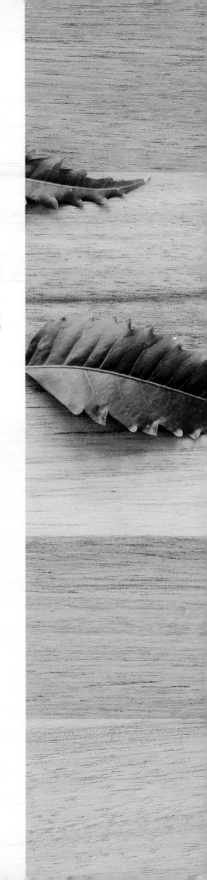

PART THREE

# DO-IT-YOURSELF HOME REMEDIES
*for*
# NATURAL HEALING

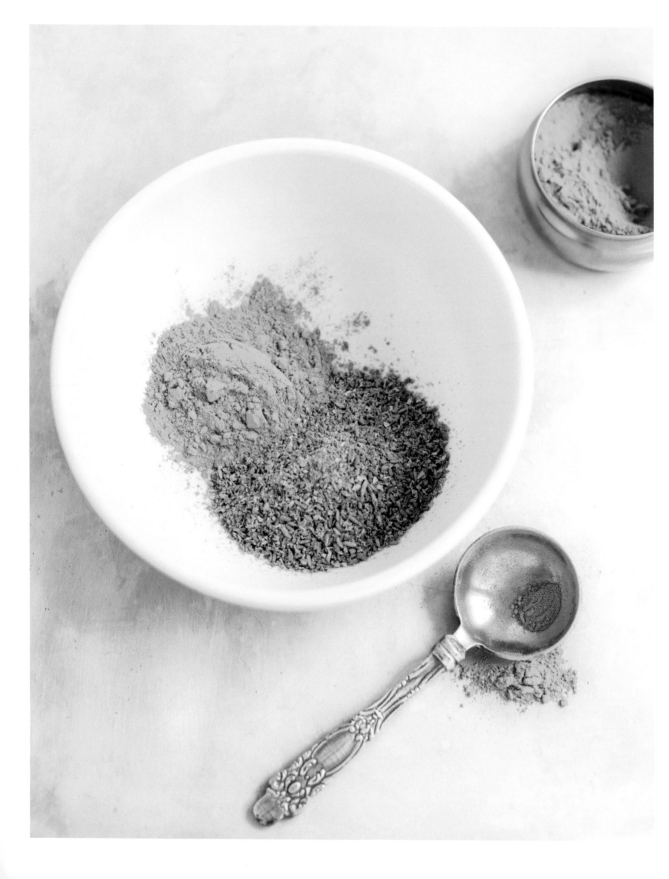

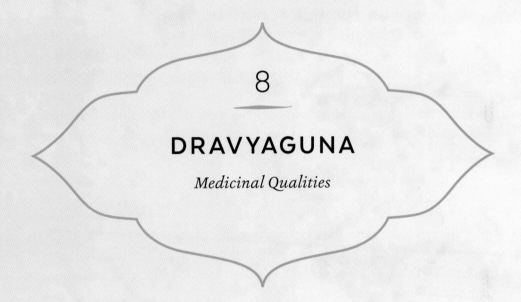

# 8

## DRAVYAGUNA

*Medicinal Qualities*

*D*ravyaguna is the science of understanding the properties and effects, both beneficial and harmful, of substances. This in-depth knowledge allows you to use foods, spices, and herbs as medicines. Ultimately, any substance is the result of its elemental constitution. The elements lend their qualities to the substance, and when that food, spice, or herb is digested, those qualities will affect the body. Many factors about the body, timing, and agni must be taken into account. The fundamental knowledge of a substance's effects is still subject to the circumstances surrounding its use. For example, penicillin is a cure for strep throat–unless a person is allergic to it, and then it can be deadly.

All of the words and concepts in this section are going to show up in the directory of spices and herbs, as well as in the remedies. I hope they help you understand more deeply how Ayurveda works, if not through reading, then through application, keen observation, and experience. Rather than blindly reaching for a tablet or tea, begin to think broadly about your symptom(s), about the current state of your body, about plausible causes, and about the effects associated with potential remedies. This knowledge will make you a more effective self-healer.

## THE FIVE ASPECTS OF A MEDICINAL SUBSTANCE

The Charaka Samhita describes a substance as a piece of cloth and the qualities and actions of that substance as the threads woven together to make the cloth. It is one thing to say ginger is good for colds and quite another to understand how, why, and when ginger is helpful. This knowledge of how a substance works has five aspects to it: *rasa, guna, virya, vipaka,* and *prabhava*.

### Rasa (Taste)

If you are into Ayurvedic cooking, you have heard of *shad rasa*, the six tastes. Each of these tastes is the result of a combination of two elements and their qualities. The taste buds perceive the elemental composition of a substance. The six tastes are sweet (*madhura*), sour (*amla*), salty (*lavana*), pungent (*katu*), bitter (*tikta*), and astringent (*kashaya*).

+ **Sweet:** Made up of earth and water, sweet is found in substances that are heavy, oily, sticky, and cool, such as bananas, milk, almonds, and rice. Sweet taste builds tissues and is especially good for the bones, skin, hair, and reproductive tissues, but in excess it can cause weight problems (a buildup of fat tissue) and diabetes. It is the most nourishing of the six tastes.
+ **Sour:** Made up of earth and fire, sour is found in substances that are heating, heavy, and moist, such as sour cream, sharp cheeses, unripe and most citrus fruits, ferments,

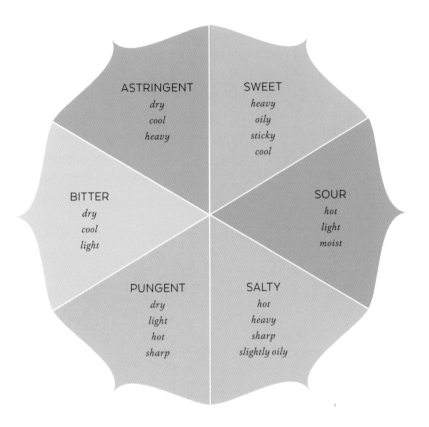

and vinegar. Sour taste increases agni and cleanses and energizes the body's tissues and senses due to its light quality. In excess, the heat and wet of sour can cause irritation and swelling.

- **Salty:** Made up of fire and water, salty is found in substances that are hot, heavy, and sharp such as sea salt, rock salt, seaweed. Salty taste holds moisture in the body, improves digestive activity, and lubricates and clears obstructions of the digestive and other channels. In excess, too much salt can cause swelling, drying of skin, and diminishing strength.

- **Pungent:** Made up of fire and air, pungent is found in substances that are dry, light, and hot, such as black and hot peppers, garlic, mustard, and onion. Pungent taste increases heat and cooks out impurities. It is helpful in removing mucus and drying up fat; it also dilates the channels of the body and gets things moving. In excess, the hot and sharp of pungency can irritate the stomach and overstimulate the mind, while the dry and light qualities can deplete the reproductive tissues.

- **Bitter:** Made up of space and air, bitter is found in substances that are dry, cool, and light such as coffee, dark leafy greens like kale and collards, fenugreek seed, and turmeric. Bitter taste reduces fat, manages blood sugar, cleans the blood of toxins, improves digestion, and reduces moisture. In excess, it can dry you out, make you cold, and deplete the body's energy.

- Astringent: Made up of air and earth, astringent is found in substances that are dry and have a downward-moving action that can aid in the removal of impurities. Examples are cranberries, fruit and vegetable skins, unripe banana, black tea, red wine, and honey. Astringency removes water from the body, tones any tissues that may be slack, watery, or fatty, and cleans the blood. In excess, astringency can make you stiff, constipated, and thirsty.

## Guna (Quality)

Here we refer back to our discussion of qualities and the five elements in chapter 1. While a substance may be sweet, it may hold more qualities of earth than of water or vice versa. We know that sweet foods are heavy, oily, sticky, and/or cool, but sometimes certain qualities predominate. For example, both milk and rice are sweet, but their qualities differ. Milk is heavy and moist, while rice is light and dry. There is more water in milk than in rice. Rice is sticky, while milk is slippery. Add water to the rice and spices to the milk, and qualities change yet again.

Gunas are the physical properties of a substance, but they may not always have the expected effects on the body. Much of the knowledge of a substance's actions comes from thousands of years of experience, and observation has led to three more aspects to consider: virya, vipaka, and prabhava. This is where it gets a little more involved.

Taking care to balance the elements in the body by enjoying a ratio of mostly sweet taste in the form of complex carbohydrates and proteins, with the addition of the other five in smaller amounts, keeps the doshas balanced and the body in equilibrium. When things are out of whack, the stronger effects of herbs and medicinal spices may be judiciously used to bring things back into balance. The taste a substance has on the tongue, in this case, is only the tip of the iceberg. What happens once it passes through the mouth and into the digestive process?

## Virya (Potency)

A substance's potency is the effect it has on the digestive tract after it is swallowed and once it has interacted with digestive enzymes. This effect can be either heating or cooling. The mahasrotas (digestive tract) is responsible for the nutrition that goes into the body and cleansing of the body and all its tissues and wastes. If this channel is too hot or too cold, all sorts of things can go awry. This channel is also the home to the doshas, and hot virya will increase pitta, while cold virya may increase vata and kapha. If one of these doshas is out of balance, virya becomes even more important. Notice how the virya of some spices in chapter 9 are cooling and others, heating. Too many heating spices can aggravate pitta, so choose wisely.

Potency is, in general, the most important thing to consider about whether a substance is appropriate or not. Someone of a hot body type may go for a cleansing yet cooling plant, such as dandelion, while someone with a cold body type in need of cleansing might choose something that clears with warmth, like peppers. Substances can also be neutral or only slightly heating or cooling. These tend to be considered good for all doshas and are more likely to be recommended often and to the public, such as triphala. Self-medicating with an herb using an incorrect virya for your body can mess you up.

### Vipaka (Postdigestive Taste)

Vipaka is the converted taste of a substance after it's been metabolized. Once a substance has been processed by the digestive tract, there can sometimes be a change in its properties and an impact on the doshas and tissues, as well as on the digestive tract. Vipaka can have three different effects on the body:

1. **Sweet:** nourishing, moist effects and cooling virya. Examples are milk, ghee, and grains.
2. **Pungent:** hot, dry effects and heating virya. Examples are peppers, broccoli, and garlic.
3. **Sour:** hot, moist effects and heating virya. Examples are tomatoes, lemons, and alcohol.

Goat's milk and cow's milk have similar taste and quality; both are sweet to the tongue, moist, and heavy. But goat's milk has pungent vipaka, while cow's milk has sweet vipaka. This is because goats eat a lot of pungent plants, while cows eat sweet ones. A tonic for the reproductive organs, which like to keep cool, calls for cow's milk, not goat's milk, and this makes a big difference. In a kapha-type scenario, however, a person may not digest cow's milk well and end up feeling congested, slow, or heavy in the stomach. If this describes you, goat's milk may digest better and leave you feeling satisfied but not bogged down. The hot and dry effect of pungent vipaka balances the heavy, moist aspects of kapha.

Vipaka is knowledge for practitioners and not something to get too involved with at home. However, sometimes when an ingredient combination or food-combining rule doesn't quite match up, it's likely due to the converted taste of a substance, as in the preceding example of goat's milk. Now it finally makes sense why goat's milk is easier to digest for those who can't tolerate cow's milk!

### Prabhava (Special Power)

Prabhava is a specific action that cannot be explained by a substance's other classifications. I think of it as a "special power." *Prahbha* means "shining light from the moon," and a substance's mystical ability to defy logic is one of my favorite things about dravyaguna. This action may actually contradict what is expected. For example, ghee is heavy and oily, but it increases agni, like lighter fluid, and does not aggravate pitta. Honey should be cooling like other sweet vipaka substances, but it is actually heating and reduces mucus; hence, it is the best sweetener for kapha and a go-to for cold remedies. Ginger tastes and feels spicy in the mouth and stomach but has a sweet aftereffect and generally does not increase heat in the body or aggravate pitta.

In modern medicine, there continue to be healing journeys that don't make sense according to Western science. Thank goodness! While figuring things out is something humans do best, reminders that dimensions of experience beyond mental understanding exist and affect us keep it real. Curiosity, hope, and healing require as much heart as they do mind.

## KARMA

Karma means action and implies reaction as well. The karma of a substance is the expected action it has on the body when used therapeutically. These actions include burning ama, kindling agni, improving absorption, promoting fertility, building tissue, and reducing mucus, to name a few. Unlike prabhava, karmas are expected. A body will have a reaction to a substance with specific results. If the substance is heating, the body will get hotter. It's undeniable, as all karmas are, like the arc of a boomerang on its course.

For example, eggplant has an *anulomina* action, which means it promotes downward movement. It can be helpful for instigating menstruation and relieving constipation. Black pepper is very sharp and heating, and its action is deepana, or kindling digestive fire. Most pungent substances have this action. Honey has a scraping action, and its karma is removing fat and mucus—it cuts sticky stuff. Rosemary stimulates circulation and improves memory with sharp and penetrating qualities; milk improves fertility by nourishing reproductive tissue with heavy, oily, cool qualities.

## HERBAL PREPARATIONS

The way a substance is processed and administered can change its qualities and its actions on the body. For example, the same herb taken as a tea, in an herbal wine, or in a medicated milk will have very different qualities: tea is light, wine is sharp, and milk is cool.

Depending on your body, the season, and the desired effect, a substance can be tailored by carefully considering the type of preparation that will be most beneficial.

## Types of Preparations

There are many kinds of herbal preparations, including tinctures, infusions, herbal wines and jams—even suppositories. The following list includes only those featured in this book. While traditional Ayurvedic medicinal formulas are quite detailed, I've focused on methods of preparation that are simple enough to do at home. The best remedy is the one you actually use!

> Churna: powdered form of a dried herb. A fresh herb such as rosemary or thyme from your garden can be dried, then ground to a powder and saved in a glass jar. The ground turmeric you buy for cooking is a *churna*. Many Ayurvedic herbal mixtures are sold as churnas already. Dry roasting spices and grinding them will yield a churna to be used for medicinal cooking.
>
> Decoction: an herb boiled in water for one or more hours to reduce and thicken the liquid. This yields a stronger product that can be taken in amounts of 1–2 tablespoons mixed with hot water.
>
> Ghrita: herbal ghee. A decoction is mixed with ghee and cooked until all the water evaporates, leaving the medicine in the ghee to form the *ghrita*.
>
> Herbal water: water in which spices or herbs are steeped or boiled for 10–20 minutes. It is brewed weak and used in large amounts, often throughout the day. It can be served hot, at room temperature, or cool, depending on the season.
>
> Infusion: a plant is steeped in hot water, covered, for 30 minutes or more.
>
> Kashayam: a strong tea. Herbs or spices are boiled in water for 5–10 minutes to yield the kashayam.
>
> Medicated milk: Powdered herbs are simmered in milk over low heat for 5–10 minutes.
>
> Thailam: herbal oil. A decoction is mixed with a base oil and simmered until the water evaporates, leaving the medicine in the oil. Plain sesame, coconut, castor, and sunflower oils are most often used to make thailam.
>
> Tincture: a cold infusion in which alcohol is used instead of water to draw the medicines out of the plant. Used for plants that are heat sensitive.

## Anupana

In dravyaguna, the preparation of a substance determines its actions. For instance, the state of the agni affects how a remedy digests. An infusion is easier to digest than a dry powder, while an herbal ghee is heavier and requires stronger agni. Digestive remedies and remedies for the superficial tissues will generally be lighter, and those for the bones, nerves, and brain will be nourishing and often contain some kind of fat. Remedies for the blood can be cleansing or nourishing but are often cooling.

Depending on what part of the body (or mind) you are trying to heal, herbs have specific substances for delivery called *anupana*. Think of these carriers as catalytic agents. Taking an herb in plain water may not do anything, while taking it in aloe or honey could be essential. This information is integrated into the home remedy recipes and explains why the combinations are important.

*Hot water* is best for rasa dhatu and fat tissue.

Nourishing *cow's milk* is best for rasa dhatu, bones, and reproductive tissues. Those who don't tolerate dairy well can use homemade *almond milk*.

*Aloe* is best for rakta dhatu and reproductive tissues where there is excessive heat.

*Honey* penetrates the muscle and fat tissues and is often used to carry herbs for reducing cholesterol and weight.

*Ghee* is ideal for soothing nerve tissue and carries nerve tonics deep into the body and brain.

### Timing

As always in Ayurveda, timing is important. While the science of timing can get very specific, here are a few important concepts for the home apothecary:

- Taking a preparation *before a meal* kindles agni and gets the fires going.
- Taking a preparation *after a meal* improves its digestion in the stomach, which in turn will improve the assimilation of nutrients.
- Preparations taken *at bedtime* improve sleep, and in some cases, create an effect the next morning, as in the case of remedying constipation.
- Preparations for detoxification are most effective when taken *first thing in the morning*.

Don't be overwhelmed! It may take some time for all of the ways of using herbs and spices therapeutically to sink in. You will find more information about how and when to use each recipe in chapter 10. The best information is the kind you gain through your own experiments. Check out the qualities of a spice or an herb in the chapter that follows, try it in one of the recipes, and see how it makes you feel. Everything you need to get started is here.

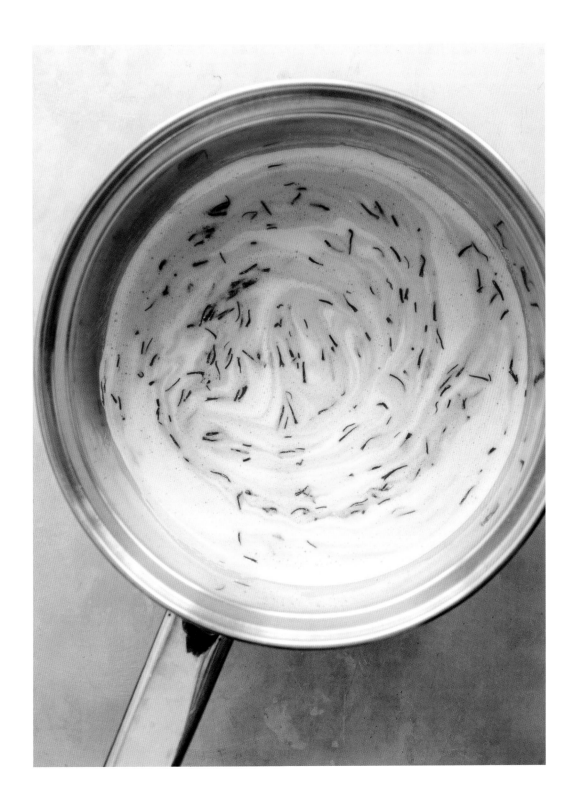

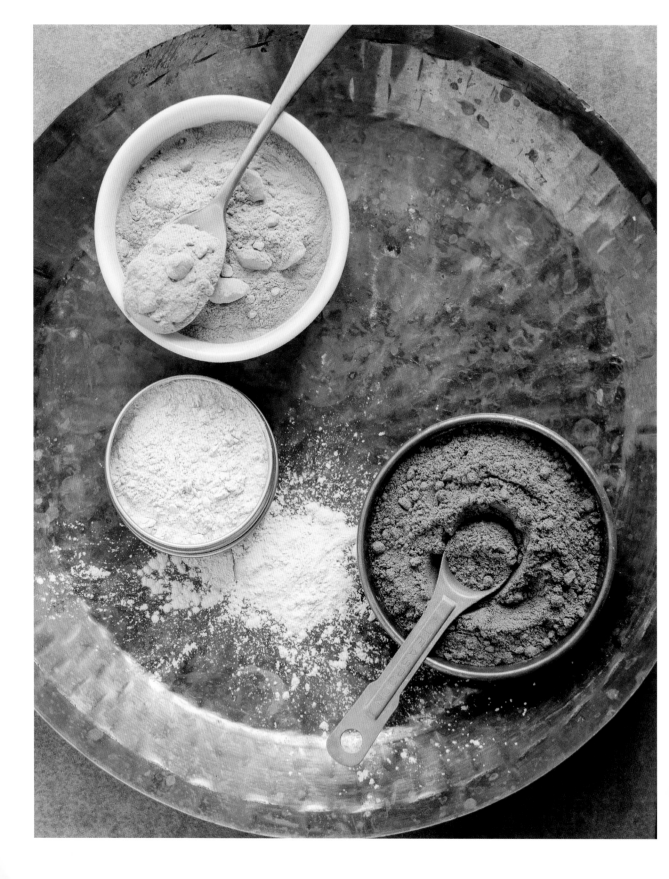

# 9

## DIRECTORY OF MEDICINAL SUBSTANCES AND HOW TO USE THEM

This directory includes mostly common kitchen spices, which are, along with healthy lifestyle, Ayurveda's most important tool for daily disease prevention. I have also included ten commonly used medicinal herbs, which are plants, like spices, but with concentrated qualities. For instance, dandelion leaves taste bitter, but they're nothing compared to the face-twisting bite of the bright green neem leaf.

You will find all of the following substances featured in the home remedies in chapter 10. The pharmacology of Ayurveda is massive, and many of the classical herbal preparations are not available outside India. I've chosen to include kitchen spices that are easy to find and likely already in your cabinet. Herbs and spices that are native to your home climate have their own qualities and healing actions. I've included a handful of North American herbs. To classify your local plants requires repeated experimentation and sensitivity to the qualities and effects these substances create in your mind and body.

## KITCHEN SPICES

### Ajwain

Ajwain looks a bit like caraway and has similar aroma and properties to thyme. It's an exotic, exciting flavor in cooking and makes a simple tea to ease a stomachache from over-indulgence. It has qualities much like those of celery seed, so if you don't have ajwain for cooking, you can substitute celery seed.

BOTANICAL NAME: *Trachyspermum ammi*

ALSO KNOWN AS: bishop's weed, *ajamoda*

PARTS USED: seeds

RASA: pungent

VIRYA: heating

VIPAKA: pungent

QUALITIES: sharp, penetrating

ACTIONS: kindles agni, improves digestion, relieves congestion

CONTRAINDICATIONS: can aggravate pitta if used regularly

Get cooking! To learn more ways to use spices as medicine in your everyday cooking, please check out *The Everyday Ayurveda Cookbook: A Seasonal Guide to Eating and Living Well.*

## Bay Leaf

This is a common Western culinary spice, made famous by Old Bay Seasoning, that is used in many kitchens to flavor meat and vegetables. It's a powerhouse that brings a trio of balancing tastes to your meals. Don't forget to pull the leaf out of the stew if you are cooking with bay leaf—you aren't supposed to eat it, and it won't soften with cooking.

BOTANICAL NAME: *Laurus nobilis* (bay laurel)

PARTS USED: leaves

RASA: pungent, bitter, sweet

VIRYA: heating

VIPAKA: pungent

QUALITIES: sharp, penetrating

ACTIONS: increases agni, improves digestion, is a decongestant (dilates the bronchi and increases airflow to the lungs); good for coughs, colds, and bronchitis

## Black Pepper

I am always asking for the pepper with a large or complicated meal. I don't bother with the usual pepper shaker and go for the fresh ground instead. I'm sure you can notice the difference in pungency! It may seem like a common substance, but do not underestimate the power of pepper. And don't skimp on your peppercorns—buy the highest quality.

BOTANICAL NAME: *Piper nigrum*

PARTS USED: seeds

RASA: pungent

VIRYA: heating

VIPAKA: pungent

QUALITIES: sharp, dry, light

ACTIONS: kindles agni; improves digestion, absorption, and elimination; increases circulation; reduces congestion

CONTRAINDICATIONS: can increase stomach acidity if taken on an empty stomach; can be drying if used in excess

*Note:* See Trikatu under "Herbs" on page 156 for Ayurveda's most common compound using black pepper.

# Cayenne/Chili

Cayenne is a variety of hot pepper, but the name is often used to describe hot pepper in general. Red chili powder and cayenne can be used interchangeably, but remember: chili powder, a mix of spices, is different from powdered red chilies.

BOTANICAL NAME: *Capsicum annuum*

ALSO KNOWN AS: red chili powder, red pepper flakes (Although cayenne is a variety of chili, "red chili" can mean many different levels of heat.)

PARTS USED: fruit, seeds

RASA: pungent

VIRYA: pungent

VIPAKA: pungent

QUALITIES: sharp, penetrating

ACTIONS: kindles agni, improves digestion, induces sweating, kills worms

CONTRAINDICATIONS: can cause diarrhea and/or irritation of the gastrointestinal tract if used in excess or in sensitive individuals

# Cardamom

A necessity for chai, green cardamom pairs well with sweets and spiced milk. I keep both the green pods and ground cardamom around, depending on whether I'm cooking with it or making teas. This spice has a broad range of healing actions and is used in many preparations.

BOTANICAL NAME: *Elettaria cardamomum*

PARTS USED: seeds

RASA: sweet, slightly pungent

VIRYA: cooling

VIPAKA: pungent

QUALITIES: light, dry

ACTIONS: increases agni; improves digestion; is used as an anti-inflammatory, aphrodisiac, and expectorant; relieves nausea

*Tip:* For nausea or bad breath, chew on a pod after meals.

## Cinnamon

There is a lot of subpar cinnamon out there, and there is no substitute for fresh cinnamon. Go the extra mile and look for strong color and aroma in ground cinnamon. Taste a pinch; it should feel pungent on your tongue. You can grind your own cinnamon sticks, but you must have a very strong grinder. An affinity for the lungs gives cinnamon a special place in cough remedies and cold medicines.

BOTANICAL NAME: *Cinnamomum zeylanicum*
PARTS USED: bark
RASA: pungent, slightly sweet, and bitter
VIRYA: heating
VIPAKA: pungent
QUALITIES: light, dry, sharp
ACTIONS: kindles agni, burns ama, improves digestion, warms the lungs, regulates blood sugar, satisfies sweet cravings, relieves dry mouth

## Cloves

Cloves are the aromatic flower buds of a tree native to Indonesia. While the majority of the global crop is used for clove cigarettes, cloves' wide range of medicinal uses has made them a regular in home remedies in many cultures. They are the first ingredient in "thieves oil," which is used to kill germs and increase immunity. Its name originates from a story of four thieves who robbed infected corpses during the bubonic plague without contracting the disease.

BOTANICAL NAME: *Eugenia caryophyllata*
PARTS USED: buds
RASA: pungent, slightly bitter
VIRYA: heating
VIPAKA: sweet
QUALITIES: penetrating
ACTIONS: increases agni, improves digestion, is an analgesic, as an oil is especially useful for gums and toothache

## Coriander

Coriander and cilantro are different parts of the same plant. Their classification is the same, but the seed's medicinal capacity is much stronger. Cilantro leaf is used all the time in Ayurvedic cooking to cool and add color. The seed is often the main ingredient in spice mixes.

BOTANICAL NAME: *Coriandrum sativum*

ALSO KNOWN AS: cilantro

PARTS USED: seeds and leaves

RASA: pungent, astringent, sweet, bitter

VIRYA: cooling

VIPAKA: sweet

QUALITIES: dry, light

ACTIONS: improves absorption, is a diuretic, reduces burning sensations

## Cumin

Native to the Middle East and India, each cumin seed arises at the center of a fruit. These seeds warm up the gut and contain good oils and lots of iron. I've had great luck moving out congestion with a tea of fresh ginger and cumin seed.

BOTANICAL NAME: *Cuminum cyminum*

ALSO KNOWN AS: *jeera*

PARTS USED: seeds

RASA: bitter, pungent, astringent

VIRYA: heating

VIPAKA: pungent

QUALITIES: light, oily

ACTIONS: kindles agni, improves digestion, relieves gas

CONTRAINDICATIONS: can be too heating if used in excess and may cause belching

## Dandelion

A member of the daisy family, yellow dandelion wildflowers are a common sight in a North American spring. This is the time of year to use the greens and roots in culinary as well as home remedy recipes to support the body's cleansing process after winter.

BOTANICAL NAME: *Taraxacum officinale*

PARTS USED: leaves, roots

RASA: bitter, astringent

VIRYA: cooling

VIPAKA: sweet

QUALITIES: light, dry

ACTIONS: cleans the blood, is a diuretic, supports liver function

CONTRAINDICATIONS: can aggravate vata if used in excess

### Fennel

Native to the Mediterranean, fennel now grows throughout the world. It is a hardy, sweet-smelling bush that tastes like licorice. You will see the white bulbs and their feathery green tops for sale at local markets. I save the tops for making broth. Chewing on a few fennel seeds after a meal calms acidity and improves digestion. These are the sugar-coated seeds you see in Indian restaurants.

BOTANICAL NAME: *Foeniculum vulgare*

PARTS USED: seeds, bulbs

RASA: sweet, astringent

VIRYA: cooling

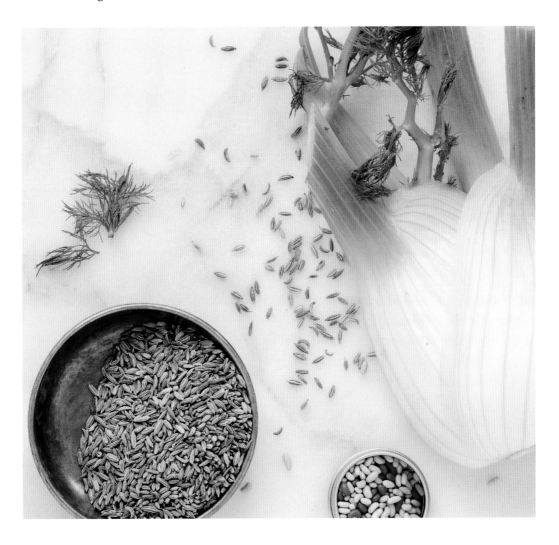

VIPAKA: sweet

QUALITIES: light

ACTIONS: tridoshic, is a blood cleanser and diuretic

*Note:* Some people cannot tolerate the taste of licorice and will reject any foods or remedies containing fennel!

## Fenugreek

Fenugreek has been used by herbalists for thousands of years. Its ability to break up blockages and move stuff out invigorates the body and assists in detoxification. It is cultivated worldwide and appears in all kinds of Eastern cooking.

BOTANICAL NAME: *Trigonella foenum-graecum*

PARTS USED: seeds

RASA: bitter, pungent

VIRYA: heating

VIPAKA: pungent

QUALITIES: dry, hot

ACTIONS: burns ama, breaks up mucus, is a diuretic and demulcent, energizes, increases the flow of breast milk

*Note:* Preparations made with this herb will make your perspiration smell like fenugreek.

## Garlic

Garlic offers five out of the six tastes, which makes it a powerful medicine for a variety of ailments. It is intensely heating, which kills germs, and is a good choice for deep winter.

BOTANICAL NAME: *Allium sativum*

PARTS USED: bulbs, scapes

RASA: sweet, salty, pungent, bitter, astringent

VIRYA: heating

VIPAKA: pungent

QUALITIES: oily, heavy

ACTIONS: is an aphrodisiac and antibacterial, increases circulation, relieves earache and other pains, lowers cholesterol

CONTRAINDICATIONS: can increase pitta, rajas, and acidity, as well as make you smelly if used in excess

## Ginger

Fresh gingerroot and ground ginger are considered different substances with different effects. Fresh ginger is very special because it increases agni without increasing the fire element in the body and is good for all body types. It is a panacea in Ayurveda. Note that fresh and dried ginger have different vipakas.

BOTANICAL NAME: *Zingiber officinale*

PARTS USED: root

RASA: pungent

VIRYA: heating

VIPAKA: sweet (fresh), pungent (dried)

QUALITIES: sharp, light

ACTIONS: increases agni, burns ama, relieves nausea, is an expectorant

CONTRAINDICATIONS: should not be consumed by people with ulcers or hemorrhoids

## Hing (Asafetida)

Hing is the resinous bark of a small tree. It can be found in powdered form, cut with wheat or fenugreek, or in crystals that dissolve when heated. This warming culinary spice is a must for bringing its oniony flavor and aroma to vegetarian dishes and to reduce gases in legumes. It appears in many herbal medicines, most often *hingvastak churna*, a compound in which it is roasted in ghee and mixed with cumin and pepper.

BOTANICAL NAME: *Ferula foetida*

PARTS USED: bark

RASA: pungent, bitter

VIRYA: heating

VIPAKA: pungent

QUALITIES: sharp, penetrating

ACTIONS: kindles agni, burns ama, reduces gas

CONTRAINDICATIONS: aggravates pitta

## Licorice

Licorice is a sweet-tasting root that can be found in powdered form and tinctures, and it is often used in teas to help chest and throat maladies. Licorice brings a good deal of moisture to the body and has a wide variety of uses, but it has an affinity for the lungs. It is especially good for dry constitutions.

BOTANICAL NAME: *Glycyrrhiza glabra*

PARTS USED: root

RASA: sweet

VIRYA: cooling

VIPAKA: sweet

QUALITIES: unctuous, heavy

ACTIONS: works as a demulcent, soothes dry throat and loosens mucus, has an affinity for the respiratory system

CONTRAINDICATIONS: can aggravate kapha and/or high blood pressure if used in excess

## Mustard Seed

The seeds of the black mustard plant are black to brown in color. Yellow mustard seeds, the ones used to make Dijon-style mustards, are milder and not used as much in Ayurvedic cooking. Mustard oil is used for cooking in cooler climates of India, and the oil can also be used topically to balance kapha.

BOTANICAL NAME: *Brassica nigra*

PARTS USED: seeds

RASA: pungent

VIRYA: heating

VIPAKA: pungent

QUALITIES: hot

ACTIONS: increases agni, burns ama, improves digestion, detoxifies

CONTRAINDICATIONS: aggravates pitta

## Nutmeg

Dried nutmeg looks a little like an avocado pit and is wonderful freshly grated onto hot cocoa or milk. It is worth keeping the whole pieces around rather than relying on the ground variety.

BOTANICAL NAME: *Myristica fragrans*

PARTS USED: fruit

RASA: bitter, astringent, pungent

VIRYA: heating

VIPAKA: pungent

QUALITIES: light, sharp

ACTIONS: kindles agni, burns ama, is used for pain relief, improves sleep

CONTRAINDICATIONS: aggravates pitta, can cause constipation if used in excess

## Peppermint

Mint is a hardy shrub known to take over gardens. It is common in most parts of the world as a digestive aid, especially for hyperacidity. Peppermint has bright green, broad leaves. Spearmint, a sharper, stronger variety, has darker, spear-shaped leaves. There are between thirteen and fifteen classified varieties of mint, and most can be used interchangeably.

BOTANICAL NAME: *Mentha piperita*

PARTS USED: leaves, stems

RASA: pungent, sweet

VIRYA: cooling

VIPAKA: sweet

QUALITIES: light, dry

ACTIONS: improves digestion, detoxifies, soothes and cools, relieves bloating

## Pippali

Known in the West as "long pepper," pippali tastes like a mild black pepper. The peppercorns are long, not round, like tiny pinecones. This dried fruit is more likely to show up in herbal medicines than in your dinner, but I do keep a grinder of pippali on the table in springtime. Its special power lies in its pungent taste but sweet aftereffect, like gingerroot, which helps to burn ama without causing an imbalance in any body type. It also has an affinity for the lungs. I go for this one first when I have a cold because I can take a lot of it without getting an acid stomach, unlike black pepper and cayenne.

BOTANICAL NAME: *Piper longum*

ALSO KNOWN AS: long pepper

PARTS USED: fruit

RASA: pungent

VIRYA: heating

VIPAKA: sweet

QUALITIES: light, sharp, dry

ACTIONS: relieves congestion, is an expectorant, increases agni, burns ama

CONTRAINDICATIONS: should not be used by people with ulcers

## Rosemary

Rosemary is an evergreen shrub in the mint family. It grows easily in all sorts of climates, but it prefers cool weather and has a wide range of benefits. Fresh is best, and this one grows great even potted indoors.

BOTANICAL NAME: *Rosmarinus officinalis*

PARTS USED: needles, stems

RASA: pungent, bitter, astringent

VIRYA: heating

VIPAKA: pungent

QUALITIES: sharp

ACTIONS: improves digestion and circulation, is a decongestant

## Saffron

Saffron is a high-antioxidant, rare floral species originating in Greece. It does not grow in the wild and thrives in warm climates. Saffron has long been prized in Eastern cultures for its rich color and aroma, as well as for its many therapeutic benefits for the skin, mind, and digestion.

BOTANICAL NAME: *Crocus sativus*

PARTS USED: flowers

RASA: astringent, bitter, sweet

VIRYA: heating

VIPAKA: pungent

QUALITIES: light, dry

ACTIONS: tridoshic, kindles agni, improves digestion, burns ama, purifies and nourishes the blood, calms the nerves

*Tip:* For a beautiful treat, try my Saffron Lassi recipe from *The Everyday Ayurveda Cookbook*.

## Salt, Mineral

Mineral salt comes from the earth, as opposed to the sea, and contains trace minerals. This salt is favored in Ayurveda because it does not heat the body as much as table salt and does not cause water retention.

ALSO KNOWN AS: pink salt, rock salt, Himalayan salt

RASA: salty

VIRYA: heating

VIPAKA: sweet

QUALITIES: heavy

ACTIONS: increases agni, improves digestion, maintains electrolyte balance, grounds the body

CONTRAINDICATIONS: should be used sparingly with pitta and kapha constitutions

## Thyme

In the mint family, thyme is an aromatic evergreen shrub that has been used in Europe for millennia. Today it is used in natural housecleaning products for its antimicrobial, antifungal properties. Fresh thyme is recommended over dried to retain the efficacy of its therapeutic oils. Try it cooked with eggs!

BOTANICAL NAME: *Thymus vulgaris*
PARTS USED: stems, leaves
RASA: pungent, astringent
VIRYA: heating
VIPAKA: pungent
QUALITIES: sharp
ACTIONS: aids digestion and circulation, energizes, has antimicrobial/antifungal properties

## Turmeric

Useful internally and topically for the skin, turmeric has countless health applications, including increasing circulation and reducing inflammation. It is most potent when cooked and used as a tea or decoction.

BOTANICAL NAME: *Curcuma longa*
PARTS USED: roots
RASA: bitter, pungent
VIRYA: heating
VIPAKA: pungent
QUALITIES: light, hot, dry
ACTIONS: tridoshic, is an anti-inflammatory, relieves indigestion, thins the blood and improves circulation, has an affinity for joints, can be used in skin tonics

## HERBS

The concentrated effects of herbs make them more likely to cause imbalances. When in doubt, use under the guidance of an Ayurvedic practitioner. I have listed twelve introductory Ayurvedic herbs that are commonly used as part of a conscious diet and lifestyle regimen to assist when early signs and symptoms arise. But take care: using herbs to make up for nonbeneficial food and lifestyle choices will only get you so far. Couple herbal remedies with wise daily living, and do not use them during pregnancy. Always check in with your health care provider about unresolved imbalances.

Many of these herbs are commonly used on a seasonal basis. An herb with pungent virya will be heating and therefore most balancing in winter and spring weather. Cooling herbs are best for warmer weather. For instance, aloe vera is cooling and often recommended in summer to pacify pitta, whereas ashwagandha is heating and can provide strength and immunity in cold months. It is not compulsory to use an herb to manage seasonal changes, but if signs and symptoms of aggravated dosha arise and are difficult to manage with diet and lifestyle, an herbal remedy can help you regain balance.

In general, herbal remedies should not be used for more than three to four months. Ideally, the imbalance will resolve within this time, and you can put aside the remedy. You will find ways to use each of these herbs in chapter 10.

### Aloe Vera

Aloe is often used in women's health remedies. Its Indian name means "virgin," and it is thought to bring the strength of youth to the reproductive system. *Kumari asava* is a very common fermented aloe drink used to balance menstrual problems and high pitta conditions. Aloe juice is used internally (look for "inner fillet or "inner leaf" on the label, as the skin contains potentially harmful latex), while aloe gel, familiar for sunburns, is used externally. Aloe gel is much stronger than aloe juice, but both come from the inner fillet of the leaf.

BOTANICAL NAME: *Aloe barbadensis*

AYURVEDIC NAME: kumari

PARTS USED: stems, roots

RASA: bitter, pungent

VIRYA: cooling

VIPAKA: sweet

QUALITIES: unctuous, heavy

ACTIONS: soothes and moisturizes entire gastrointestinal tract, is an anti-inflammatory and a laxative, rejuvenates, improves menstrual flow

SEASON: summer

CONTRAINDICATIONS: can cause diarrhea if used in excess, laxative effect is habit-forming with long-term use

*Note:* Aloe juice is now easy to find in gallon-size jugs or in sugar-packed green bottles near the checkout counter. The unsweetened kind makes a refreshing summer beverage but will not have the same medicinal qualities as the plant itself. Lily of the Desert and Aloe Life are trusted brands for aloe juice. See Homemade Aloe Juice on page 176.

### Amalaki

Amalaki is a powerful rejuvenating herb packed with vitamin C. It is the main ingredient in *chyawanprash*, a rasayana found in most Indian homes, and in triphala, a common digestive compound. This powder, made of the dried amla fruit, is said to enhance and preserve life and can be used by people of all ages. It tastes very sour but has a sweet aftertaste, a rare and prized combination for nourishing all the dhatus.

BOTANICAL NAME: *Emblica officinalis*

ALSO KNOWN AS: Indian gooseberry, amla, emblic

PARTS USED: fruit

RASA: sour, bitter, astringent, sweet, salty

VIRYA: cooling

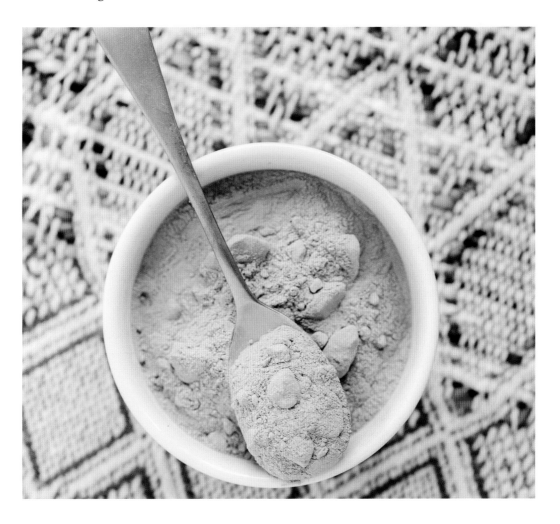

VIPAKA: sweet

QUALITIES: light

SEASON: summer, fall

ACTIONS: nourishes all seven tissues, purifies the blood, relieves acid indigestion

## Ashwagandha

The name of this herb from the Himalayan foothills means "smell of a horse." While ashwagandha does smell like a horse, its use is said to bring the strength of that animal. This is a common tonic herb for male reproductive vitality and an adaptogen, which helps the body cope with stress. It is a go-to for supporting vata constitutions.

BOTANICAL NAME: *Withania somnifera*

ALSO KNOWN AS: winter cherry

PARTS USED: roots, bark

RASA: bitter, astringent

VIRYA: heating

VIPAKA: sweet

QUALITIES: heavy, unctuous

ACTIONS: nourishes all seven tissues, improves strength and reduces fatigue, improves memory

SEASON: winter

CONTRAINDICATIONS: can aggravate pitta if used in excess

## Brahmi

Brahmi is Ayurveda's star nerve tonic, used to increase intelligence, memory, and support the nervous system. It is commonly used in the West as well, where it is known as *gotu kola*. The subtle root system resembles a brain. It's most commonly used in brahmi ghee, which targets the nerve and brain tissues.

BOTANICAL NAME: *Centella asiatica*

ALSO KNOWN AS: gotu kola, Indian pennywort

PARTS USED: leaves, branches, roots

RASA: bitter, astringent

VIRYA: cooling

VIPAKA: sweet

QUALITIES: unctuous, sharp, subtle

ACTIONS: improves memory, sleep, and mental focus

SEASON: year-round

## Castor Oil

Castor seeds are boiled to yield the thickest, heaviest oil available. Castor oil can penetrate the tissues and is used for breaking up stagnation and blockage, as well as for healing connective tissues. Externally it is a strong anti-inflammatory and pain reliever, and internally it is one of the strongest purgatives. Castor oil does wonders for softening the skin and healing scar tissue.

BOTANICAL NAME: *Ricinus communis*

PARTS USED: seeds

RASA: sweet, pungent, astringent

VIRYA: cooling (externally), heating (internally)

VIPAKA: sweet

QUALITIES: heavy, oily, dense, sharp, penetrating

ACTIONS: breaks up blockages, is a strong purgative and anti-inflammatory, induces labor and menstruation, penetrates deep tissue, relieves low backache

SEASON: summer (external use)

CONTRAINDICATIONS: ingesting castor oil can cause imbalances, so seek professional guidance before taking it

*Tip:* See the recipe for a Castor Oil Pack (page 260) for external uses.

## Lavender

Lavender, a member of the mint family, is so beloved that a color is named after the hue of its flowers. It has been used in both medicine and perfume for millennia. Common as a culinary herb and an essential oil, it is one of the Western herbs I have chosen to include because it grows easily and smells and looks wonderful in a garden. Its leaves and flowers can be used in teas and herbal honeys for relaxation and pain relief.

BOTANICAL NAME: *Lavendula angustifolia*

PARTS USED: flowers, stems, leaves

RASA: pungent, astringent

VIRYA: slightly cooling

VIPAKA: pungent

QUALITIES: dry, cold

ACTIONS: is used as a carminative, nervine sleep aid and muscle relaxant; reduces pitta

SEASON: year-round, especially summer

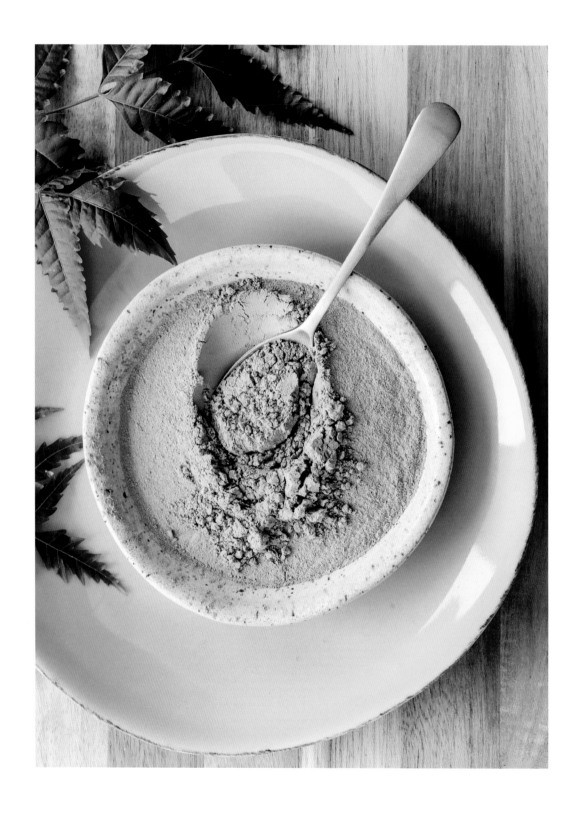

## Moringa

Moringa, whose name is derived from the Tamil "drumstick," is a common ingredient in South Indian sambar, a spicy breakfast soup. It took many years of avoiding the barked pieces in my breakfast before I learned of moringa's medicinal properties. Moringa powder, made from the dried leaves of the tree, is becoming easier to find as a mineral-rich, green superfood. Its benefits are far-reaching, and it has been shown to aid digestion and circulation. Due to its penetrating and heating qualities, it has an affinity for meda dhatu and may assist in weight loss.

BOTANICAL NAME: *Moringa oleifera*

ALSO KNOWN AS: drumstick tree, horseradish tree

PARTS USED: roots, fruit, leaves, bark

RASA: pungent, bitter

VIRYA: heating

VIPAKA: pungent

QUALITIES: light, dry, penetrating

ACTIONS: detoxifies, is good as an anti-inflammatory and for weight loss

SEASON: spring

## Neem

A common ingredient in toothpaste, twigs of the neem tree were used to clean the teeth in the days of old. Due to its intense bitterness, it is a strong antibacterial and antiparasitic. On my first trip to India, I was told to eat a few leaves daily to ward off bugs. I could barely get them down! Externally, neem oil is commonly used for skin conditions.

BOTANICAL NAME: *Azadirachta indica*

ALSO KNOWN AS: nimba

PARTS USED: flowers, fruit, leaves, bark

RASA: bitter

VIRYA: cooling

VIPAKA: pungent

QUALITIES: light, sharp

ACTIONS: reduces fevers, kills parasites, controls acne and eczema, purifies the blood

SEASON: summer

CONTRAINDICATIONS: extended or increased use can aggravate vata

## Shatavari

*Shatavari* means "woman who has one hundred husbands," implying its efficacy as a female fertility and vitality tonic. Shatavari contains estrogen precursors, which means it helps the body develop the female hormone estrogen. Heavy, moist qualities make it a calming and strengthening tonic, especially when mixed with almond or cow's milk.

BOTANICAL NAME: *Asparagus racemosus*

ALSO KNOWN AS: asparagus root

PARTS USED: roots

RASA: sweet, bitter

VIRYA: cooling

VIPAKA: sweet

QUALITIES: heavy, unctuous

SEASONS: fall and winter

ACTIONS: promotes breast health, female fertility, and vitality; calms the mind

CONTRAINDICATIONS: not to be used if you are at risk of breast cancer

## Triphala

Use of this triple-fruit compound as a digestive tonic is recommended by some Ayurvedic doctors as part of a general daily routine. The three fruits—*bibhitaki* for the stomach, amalaki for the small intestine, and *haritaki* for the colon—are dried and cooked; a powdered black ash is the final product, which is used internally as well as externally. This balanced digestive is good for all body types. Triphala also has an affinity for the eyes and skin and is used topically for wounds, hair health, and even in black *kajal* (a traditional eyeliner that tones the eyes—which is not the case in conventional eyeliners, even if they are called "kajal").

PARTS USED: fruits

RASA: all but salty

VIRYA: neutral

VIPAKA: sweet

QUALITIES: light, dry

ACTIONS: tridoshic, nourishes and tones all tissues, is a mild laxative and an antioxidant, rejuvenates

SEASON: year-round

CONTRAINDICATIONS: loses its efficacy with prolonged use; it's good to take a week off monthly, or a month off after every four

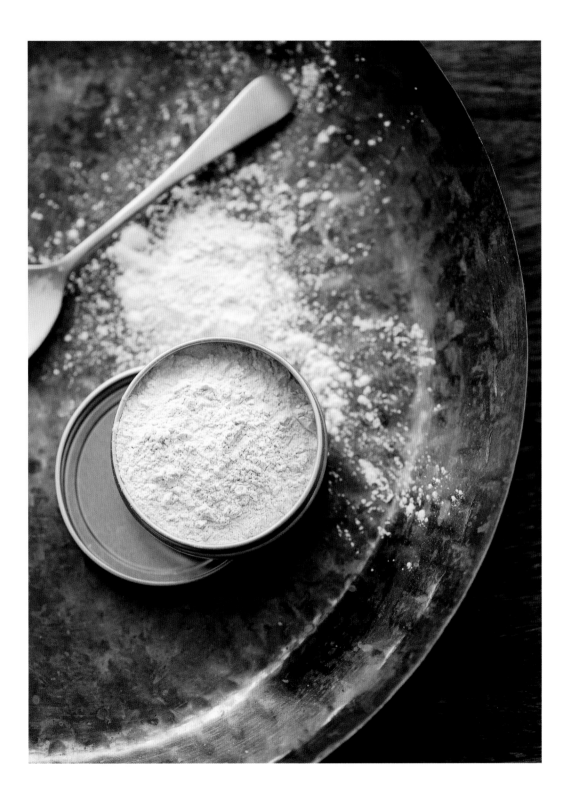

## Trikatu

*Trikatu* means "three hots" and contains equal parts ground ginger, black pepper, and pippali (long pepper). This compound is commonly used for digestive as well as respiratory ailments. A pinch is present in most herbal compounds to increase the bioavailability of the other herbs by improving digestion. It is an essential during cool, damp seasons.

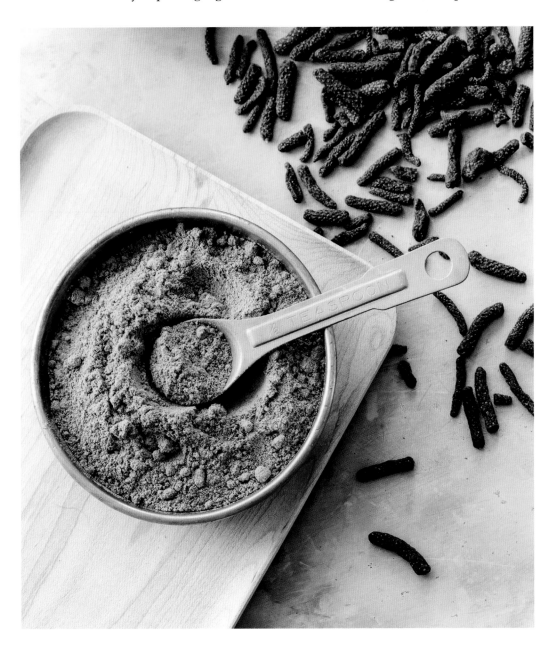

When you are cleansing or in need of a detox, take ½–1 teaspoon triphala nightly in hot water as a general health tonic. This will support your entire digestive system. While triphala's benefits can be great, I prefer to work with diet and lifestyle to preserve health and save herbal medicines for times of immediate need. I lean on triphala to ward off the dreaded travel constipation and for digestive support after indulgent meals. It's definitely in my travel kit.

PARTS USED: fruits

VIPAKA: pungent

VIRYA: heating

VIPAKA: pungent

QUALITIES: light, dry

SEASON: spring

ACTIONS: thins mucus, increases agni, is used as an expectorant

CONTRAINDICATIONS: can aggravate pitta or cause acid stomach

*Tip:* During cold and allergy season, taking ½ teaspoon of trikatu after meals twice daily helps keep your airways clear.

## Tulsi

Also called holy basil, tulsi can commonly be found as a tea in the supermarket these days. This plant has an affinity for the respiratory system and improves breathing and circulation. A great tonic for kapha, tulsi clears the mind and energizes the body. Believed to nourish the spiritual heart, tulsa is common at temples.

BOTANICAL NAME: *Ocimum sanctum*

ALSO KNOWN AS: holy basil

PARTS USED: leaves, stems

RASA: pungent, bitter

VIRYA: heating

VIPAKA: pungent

QUALITIES: subtle, light, dry

SEASON: spring

ACTIONS: stimulates circulation and detoxification, improves respiration, reduces fevers

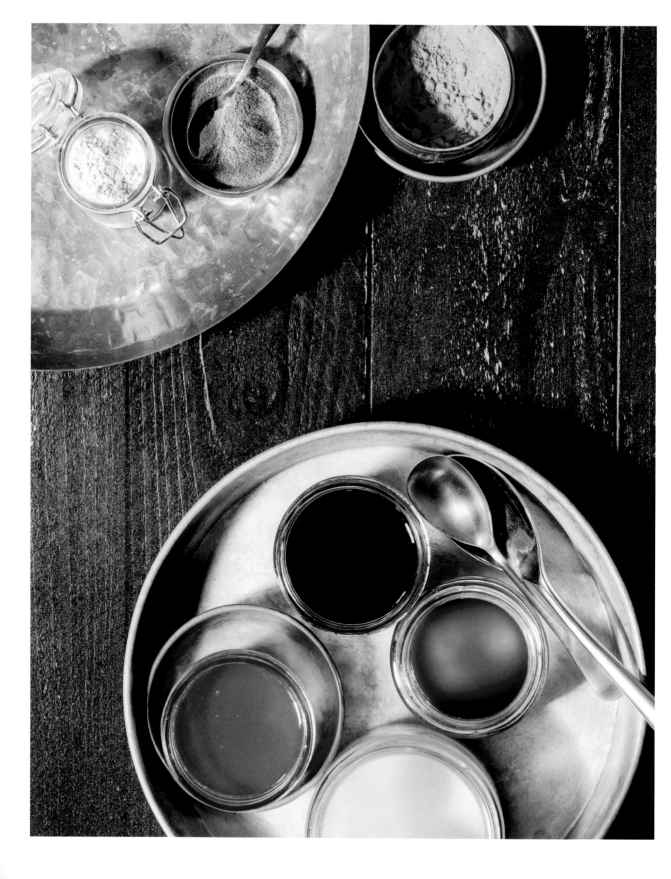

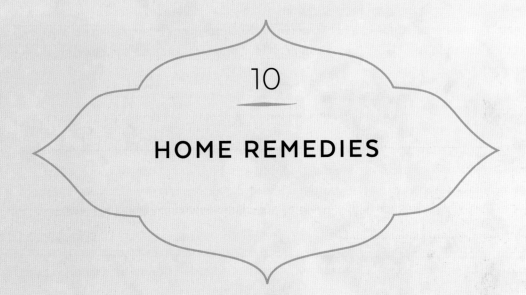

10

HOME REMEDIES

Welcome to the do-it-yourself healing recipes! I have divided the recipes into sections based on the anupana, or the carrier substance that brings therapeutic qualities into the body. These range from aloe vera juice to milks of animal and plant origins to oils, teas, honey, and ghee. Each of these carriers is meant to affect certain tissue types, or one of the doshas. I've also included a section of medicinal foods and homemade skin care products. It is likely you will find yourself drawn to a certain section, or a few sections, based on your body type, time of life, climate, and any imbalances you might be feeling. The groupings of recipes illuminate how the qualities of these substances, and their specific preparations, can help you target the cleansing or rejuvenation of the body at the right time, as well as address simple management of common ups and downs as you experience them.

## ESSENTIAL SUPPLIES

Before getting started on your healing journey in the kitchen, there are a few tools you will want to add for the simmering, straining, grating, grinding, and storing of your medicinal preparations. Check out this list before you undertake the recipes, so you have everything on hand. The right tool can be key to ease of preparation and an effective final product.

**Carafe blender:** A blender with a glass carafe has more power than a hand blender and is called for in recipes in which the ingredients are too hard or fibrous for a hand blender, such as fresh juices. A high-speed blender is great, if you have one. If not, you may have to chop vegetable stems and dates more before blending.

**Cheesecloth:** Use several layers to strain milk solids when making ghee and to strain herbs from herbal oils and ghees.

**Electric milk frother:** A small battery-operated whisk will mix powders into milk nicely and can make a little froth on top, if desired. It's ideal and quick for single-serve tonics.

**Fine mesh sieve:** A colander's holes are too big for herbal sediments, so a metal, fine mesh strainer is essential for straining. It may be used to strain the pulp from nut milks and sediment from herbal oils, as well as to separate dairy solids from ghee.

**Frying pan:** A frying pan is broad and wide, with a short lip, and is used for dry roasting, sautéing, and frying. "Green" frying pans with a ceramic nonstick covering are preferable

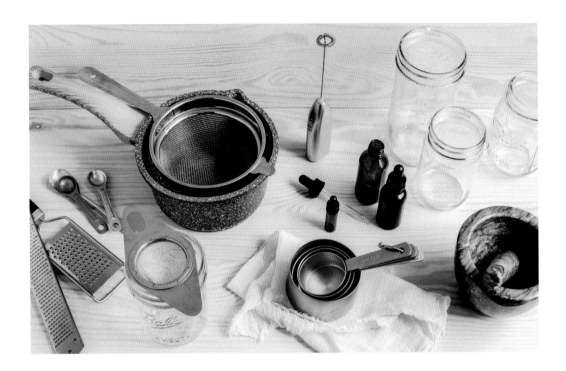

to other nonstick surfaces. Get rid of your Teflon, which can create harmful chemical compounds if the coating breaks down into your food.

**Glass water bottle:** To avoid drinking from plastic or metal all the time, using a glass water bottle for storing and transporting herbal waters is a good idea. This can be a mason jar or something fancier.

**Grater:** Metal box graters are common, but a plane grater takes up less space in the kitchen. A good grater should have small and large grating options and be sturdy. Microplane graters work great for grating gingerroot and nutmeg.

**Hand blender:** Also known as an immersion blender or stick blender, a hand blender may be used to blend nut milks and purée soups, and is quicker to clean than a carafe blender. It works especially well for single servings of takra and for hot soups, which can make a carafe too hot.

**Long-handled spoon:** Have a long-handled wooden or stainless steel spoon for stirring hot herbal oils, decoctions, and teas.

**Mason jars:** This book calls for wide-mouth, glass mason jars with lids that hold 8, 16, and 32 ounces. These can be found in the canning supplies at a hardware store and are a great way to store herbal oils, honeys, and teas. Repurposed jars with tight lids also work, but clean and dry them carefully first.

**Measuring cups and spoons:** Have a glass, 16-ounce measuring cup in your kitchen and a set of dry measuring cups as well. Keep a set of measuring spoons that range from ⅛ teaspoon to 1 tablespoon.

**Mortar and pestle:** Stone grinding is traditional in much of Ayurvedic medicine making, and it is still common to see home cooks sitting down to grind the day's ingredients. A stone mortar and pestle will not retain scents, while wood does.

**Pepper mill:** Freshly ground pepper is a joy of life. Look for a wooden pepper mill and fill it with high-quality black or multicolor peppercorns.

**Saucepans:** Look for soup pots with high walls, usually in 2-, 4-, and 6-quart sizes. A 4-quart pot is best for recipes that serve four or more, while a 2-quart pan can be used to make smaller amounts. Favor high-quality stainless steel saucepans such as All-Clad brand and do not buy aluminum, which is soft, porous, and reactive to certain foods. This can create questionable chemical compounds in your food. It is worth the investment to buy a few good saucepans.

**Spice grinder:** A coffee grinder reserved for spices, seeds, and nuts allows you to make large amounts of spice mixes quickly for storage.

**Tea strainer:** A small, fine mesh metal strainer with a handle is ideal for straining teas.

**Thermos:** A 16- or 32-ounce insulated stainless steel thermos, with a cap that doubles as a cup, can be used to store and keep hot medicinal teas for up to twelve hours. The cap will make it easy for you to drink continuously, even on the road. Splurge on a quality thermos and you won't regret it.

**Tincture bottle:** A small, 2-ounce glass dropper bottle should be brown or blue to protect the contents from light. The cap contains a dropper to be used for oiling the nose and ears.

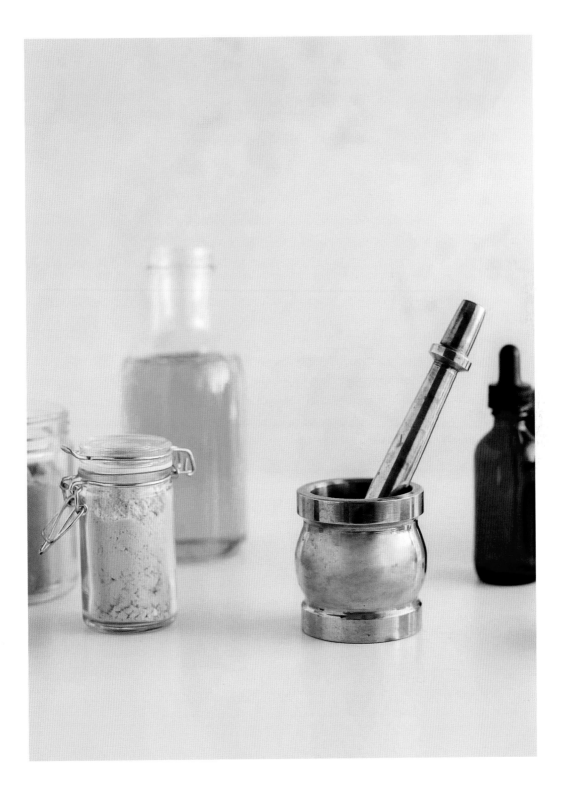

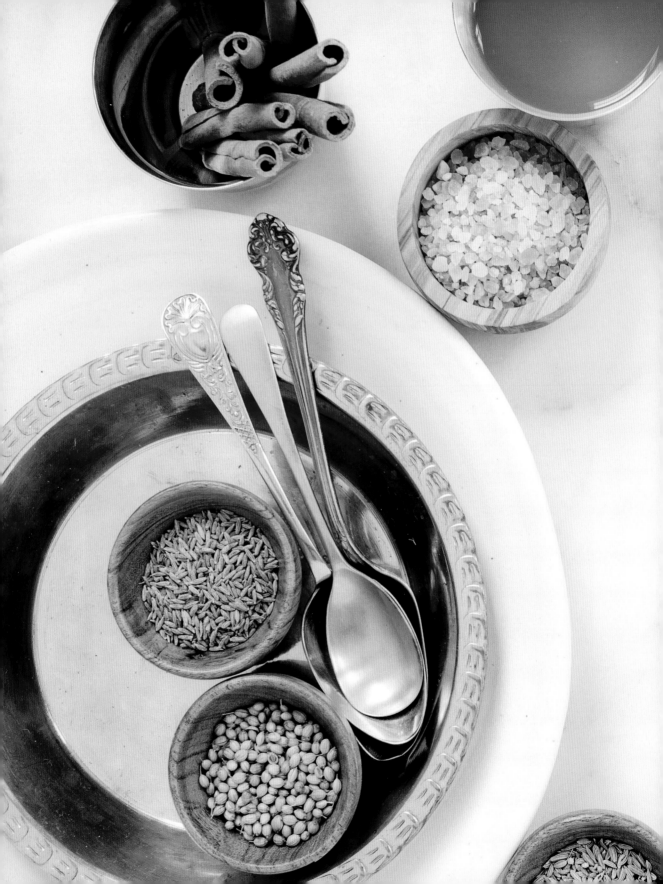

# HOME REMEDY RECIPES

The recipes in this section have been divided into ten categories to make it easier for you to find a remedy for specific situations.

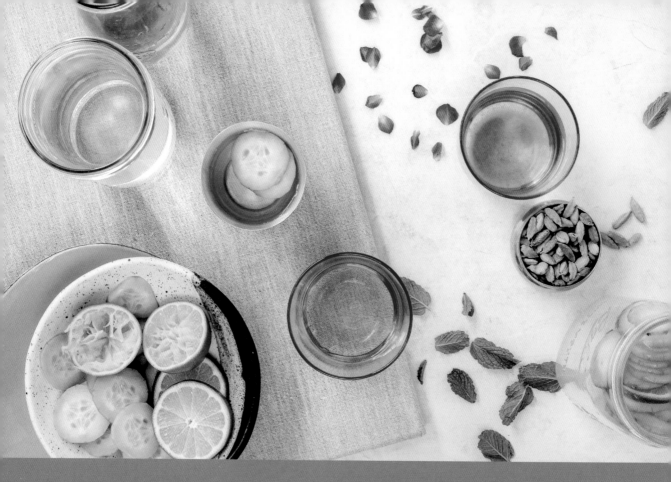

# HEALING HERBAL WATERS

The practice of drinking herbal water for health is ancient. In most areas of India, parts of local plants and trees are used for their health benefits, as well as for purification. Infusing herbs and spices into water extracts the healing oils from the plants, and the practice of hydrating with medicinal water can prevent illness, as well as reverse imbalances—even long-standing ones.

I like the healing water recipes because they are unsweetened yet tasty, simply water plus healing plants. It is important, though, not to drink these all the time but to also enjoy plain old water sometimes. During a cleanse or when I'm in need of healing, I will drink exclusively herbal water; when I'm feeling better, I will return to regular water.

Water that has been standing overnight is considered stale, and less vitalizing, so it's best to make a fresh batch each day. You may need to double the recipe. Keep it hot in a thermos or enjoy it at room temperature. Also, when using powdered spices, take care that they are fresh, or else they will have far fewer medicinal properties. Buy only the amount you need to avoid wasting any precious plants.

# BASIC COOKED WATER

*MAKES 1½-2 QUARTS*   When you have that heavy feeling in your gut or your mind, make a day's batch of cooked water and consume only that until you feel better. Drink it at a temperature that balances your environment—so warm/hot in wintertime and cool in summer.

2 qts water

In a large saucepan, bring water to a boil.

Continue to boil, uncovered, for 5 minutes. Drink it hot, warm, or at room temperature.

*Note:* If you're dealing with water retention, excess mucus, or weak digestive fire, boil uncovered for 15-20 minutes.

## COOKED WATER

Yes, I'm serious. *Cooked water.* Water itself is considered a medicinal substance, whose qualities can be improved by processing. For example, boiling water increases its lightness and decreases its heaviness. This makes it easier to digest. The Ashtanga Hrdayam states, "Water which has been boiled then cooled will not increase moisture in the body." [1] If your body is heavy on the water element, you are sitting around a lot, or you are experiencing mental stagnation, drinking cooked water can result in more light qualities in digestion and in your body as a whole. I always turn to cooked water after the holidays for a week or so, when my digestion feels heavy.

# CINNAMON WATER

*MAKES 1 QUART*   Taken throughout the day, cinnamon water regulates blood sugar, controls sugar cravings, and gives a feeling of satisfaction after meals.

1 qt water

3 cinnamon sticks or 1 tbsp freshly ground cinnamon

In a medium saucepan, bring the water to a boil. Add the cinnamon sticks, and simmer for 10-15 minutes. This method will make your house smell nice.

If using ground cinnamon, add it to the boiling water. Remove from the heat and steep for 20 minutes.

For both methods, pour the liquid through a tea strainer into a jar or thermos, and drink it throughout the day.

# AJWAIN WATER

***MAKES 1 QUART*** Ajwain (also called bishop's weed and carom seed) has a pungent, lively flavor similar to caraway and is used for a host of benefits. This herbal water, also known as *oma* water, is slightly heating and removes mucus from the body, which can help to relieve sinus and chest congestion, as well as constipation. It has a carminative effect and is often used for stomach or intestinal pain in both adults and children. Ajwain water can be a good choice for the common cold, indigestion, and loss of appetite when there is a heavy feeling in the stomach. Consuming a cup of ajwain water daily may also boost metabolism.

1 tbsp ajwain seeds

1 qt water

In a pan over medium heat, dry roast the seeds until fragrant.

In a medium saucepan, bring the water to a boil. Add the seeds, cover, and simmer for about 10 minutes.

Allow the tea to cool a bit, then strain through a tea strainer into a glass jar. Drink hot or at room temperature.

# CORIANDER AND FENNEL WATER

***MAKES 1 QUART*** Health is wealth, and *dhania* (coriander) means "wealthy one." The combination of coriander and fennel is cooling, sweet, bitter, and astringent. This makes it a great tonic for detoxification and gives it digestive properties that aid in the assimilation of nutrients. You can also double the quantity of one spice and leave out the other, making simply coriander water or fennel water.

1 qt water

1 tsp coriander seed

1 tsp fennel seed

In a medium saucepan, bring the water to a boil.

Add the coriander and fennel seeds, and boil for 10–15 minutes.

Cool and strain the liquid through a tea strainer into a glass jar.

# MINT WATER

*MAKES 1 QUART* Mint is a robust herb that is easy to come by. There is an infinite variety of mints, from chocolate mint to lemon mint. Any of them will work for herbal water, and you can have fun trying different flavors. Peppermint is the closest to the mint used in Ayurvedic medicines. Mint water soothes digestion, relieves mental stress, and is a great way to stay calm and relaxed through a busy day.

1 qt water

4 sprigs fresh mint or ⅓ cup mint leaves

In a medium saucepan, bring the water to a boil.

Remove from the heat, add the mint, and cover. Steep at least 15 minutes. Allow the mint water to cool to room temperature, then pour through a tea strainer or mesh sieve into a glass jar.

# FENUGREEK WATER

*MAKES 1 QUART* Also known as *methi*, fenugreek is bitter and light, and it is used in cooking all over Asia. It is very effective at staving off and reducing water retention and bloating, as well as controlling blood sugar and supporting liver function. Women all over the world have historically used fenugreek to increase lactation. It makes a great tonic for spring. Soaking the seeds overnight gives the liquid a fine yellow hue.

1 qt water

2 tbsp fenugreek seeds

In a medium saucepan, bring the water to a boil. Add the fenugreek seeds, cover, and soak overnight.

In the morning, pour the liquid through a tea strainer into a quart-size mason jar or steel thermos and drink throughout the day.

# CUCUMBER LIME WATER

*MAKES 1 QUART*  This recipe features a cold infusion, which appeals in summer weather. Plants that are delicate do well when steeped in cold water rather than cooked. The final product will be a refreshing, cooling, and hydrating hot-weather go-to tonic that has the bonus of supporting clear skin. This is also very easy to prepare in a pitcher, so you can serve it as something special for guests.

½ small cucumber, peeled and thinly sliced

1 qt water

Juice of 1 lime

In a quart-size glass jar, submerge the cucumber in the water. Add the lime juice.

Cover tightly, shake gently, and refrigerate for 1–8 hours. Serve the water with the cucumber pieces in it, or strain them out if you won't be drinking it soon. Allow the water to warm up a bit before drinking, unless it's very hot out!

Keep refrigerated and drink within 2–3 days.

# MORINGA COCONUT WATER

*MAKES 16 OUNCES*  All hail moringa! This is a delicious and refreshing way to work Ayurveda's mineral-rich superfood into your postworkout routine. Moringa may help control blood sugar, boost weight loss, and reduce inflammation. Whip up this drink to cool down and rejuvenate after your daily exercise.

2 cups coconut water

1 tbsp moringa powder

1 cup pineapple chunks (optional)

Add the coconut water and moringa powder to a bottle or jar with a tight lid and shake. Serve immediately.

If using pineapple, mix all the ingredients in a blender on high speed for 1 minute.

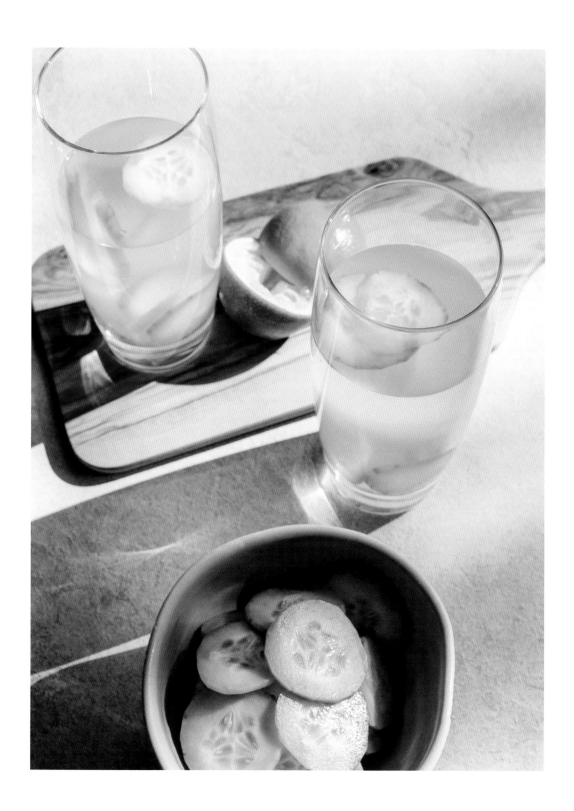

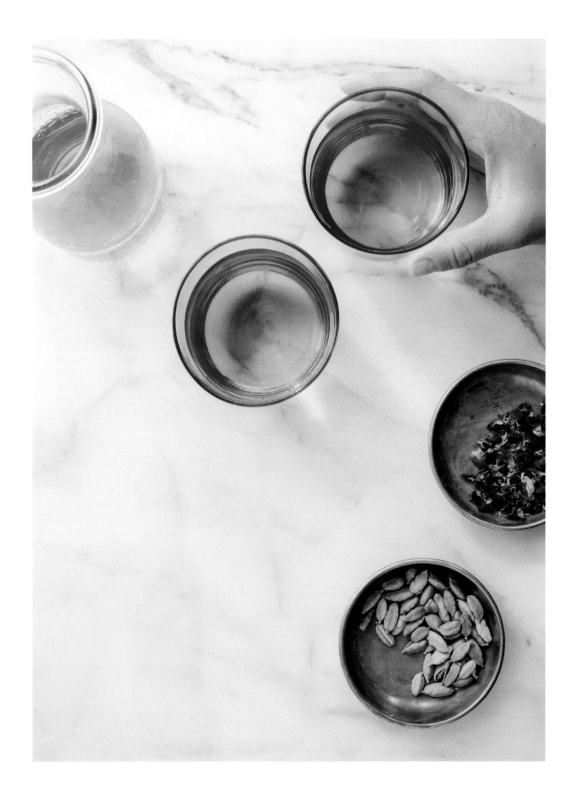

# CARDAMOM WATER

*MAKES 1 QUART*  Another refreshing and hydrating spiced drink for warm weather, cardamom water boosts metabolism, freshens the breath, and alkalizes the body. I find this one especially nice when I get tired of drinking regular water. If you come across food-grade dried rose petals, scoop them up and add a tablespoon to make cardamom rose water for a treat.

| | |
|---|---|
| 1 qt water | In a medium saucepan, bring the water to a boil. |
| 7–8 green cardamom pods | Crack open the cardamom pods in a mortar and pestle, or by crushing them with the back of a serving spoon. |
| | Add the pods to the water and simmer for 15 minutes. Let cool and strain the liquid into a glass jar. |

# TULSI WATER

*MAKES 1 QUART*  Tulsi (holy basil) has antibacterial and antifungal properties that ward off the common cold. Taken as herbal water, it has diuretic properties, detoxifies the kidneys, controls fever, and improves circulation.

| | |
|---|---|
| ¼ cup dried tulsi or 10–12 fresh tulsi leaves | Place the tulsi in a heat-safe vessel for steeping. A saucepan with tight lid or a mason jar will do. |
| 1 qt water | In a medium saucepan, bring the water to a boil. Pour it over the tulsi, cover tightly, and steep for at least 20 minutes. |
| | Pour the tulsi tea through a tea strainer into another jar or thermos and drink throughout the day. |

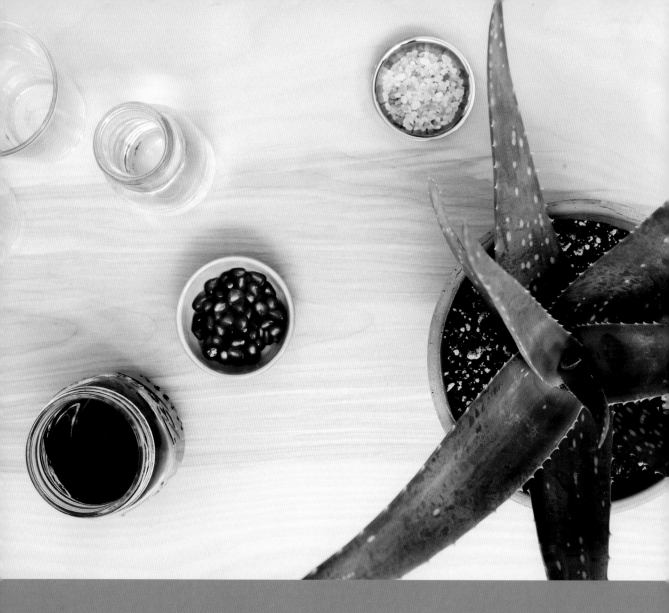

# ALOE COOLERS

*Kumari*, the Sanskrit word for the aloe plant, comes from the root for "virgin," or young girl, and speaks to its importance as a youth-giving tonic. Its bitter taste brings a cooling effect to the body and makes aloe a traditional carrier substance for herbal medicines to cool the reproductive tissues. Consuming aloe, even alone, can nourish and cool tissues, promoting a sense of calm, improved fertility, and regular menstruation. Aloe also soothes and cools the stomach, small intestine, and skin.

# ALOE CRANBERRY COOLER

*MAKES 12 OUNCES*  Heat caused by internal factors such as hormonal changes, pitta imbalances, or stress can result in urinary tract imbalances. The first sign is what I call "hot pee." This usually occurs in extremely hot weather, after heated exercise sessions, or when the body is becoming dehydrated. The next sign is difficulty peeing. Noticing an increase in the temperature of your urine can help you head off imbalance at the pass by hydrating and slowing down, perhaps with a tall one of these. It's likely you have already heard of cranberry's ability to cleanse the urinary channel. In Ayurveda we chalk this up to the fruit's astringency, a combination of earth and air elements that pulls liquid down and out.

½ cup pure
cranberry juice

½ cup aloe juice

½ cup water

2 tsp raw honey,
dissolved in warm
water (optional)

Mix the cranberry juice, aloe juice, and water together in a mason jar.

Drink a 4-oz glass after each meal, one to three times a day, at room temperature. In hot weather, you can also enjoy a cool cup anytime.

*Note:* You will find pure cranberry juice in a quart-size glass jar at most grocery stores; the most common brand is Knudsen's. This is not in the refrigerator section. If you can source fresh, local cranberries, make your own!

# HOMEMADE ALOE JUICE

*MAKES 1 CUP*  Aloe is a great plant that requires little care and grows easily. If you live in a colder climate, keep one in your house and repot it every few years. Your home-remedy garden indoors! Take care not to get any green skin in your gel, as it may cause diarrhea. This juice is the basis for all the aloe cooler recipes.

**2 tbsp aloe gel (from 1 aloe vera leaf)**

**1 cup water**

Rinse the aloe vera leaf well and pat dry.

Starting at the juicy end (not the pointy end) of the leaf, slit the skin with a paring knife and peel open the outer layer.

Scoop off the clear gel with a small spoon and put in blender carafe or wide-mouth jar. Discard the green skin.

Add the water to the aloe gel. Using a hand blender or carafe blender, blend the mixture on high. It will create a latte-like foam.

Drink immediately, or keep it for 1 week in the refrigerator.

*Note:* If you find this too bitter or experience loose stools, reduce the amount of aloe gel by half.

For a salty/sweet/bitter hydrator: Add a few cucumber slices for cucumber aloe juice, or a pinch of pink salt and 2 tsp evaporated cane juice.

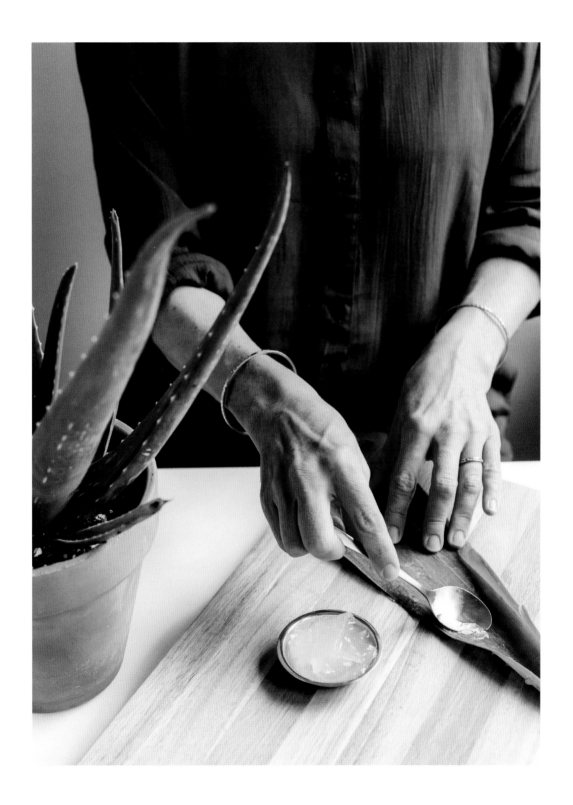

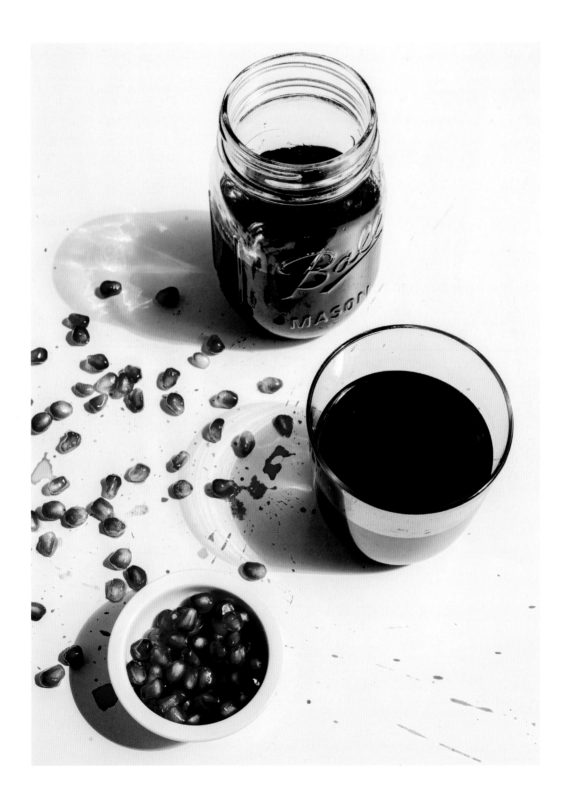

# ALOE POMEGRANATE COOLER

*MAKES 16 OUNCES*  This mixture of cooling aloe and purifying pomegranate is helpful for maintaining a regular and comfortable menstrual cycle. Its affinity for the blood makes it a good choice for skin rashes and pimples as well.

1 cup pure
pomegranate juice
(preferably fresh)

½ cup aloe juice

½ cup water

Mix the pomegranate juice, aloe juice, and water together in a mason jar. Drink a 4-oz glass after each meal, one to three times a day, at room temperature. In hot weather, you can also enjoy a cool cup anytime.

## SIGNS OF HEAT IN THE MENSTRUAL CYCLE

Ladies, these signs can alert you that you need this remedy to help you cool down and enjoy an easier time of it during your monthly cycle.

- Headaches
- Pimples
- Cramping
- More than five days of heavy menstrual flow

# KATE'S BEACH DRINK 1, 2, AND 3

I know it's not great for me, but I love sunbathing. I love the beach and the feeling of warm sand and warm sun, but too much sun and I feel overheated, weak, and tired, even the next day. To avoid accumulating too much heat, I bring a quart of cool aloe tonic in an insulated flask with me to the beach, along with a bag of red grapes. I suggest you do the same! These drinks are also great after sweating or when you start to feel that plain water isn't doing enough to quench your thirst.

### BASIC BEACH DRINK  *MAKES 1 QUART*

1 cup aloe juice

3 cups water

Combine the aloe juice and water in a 1-qt insulated water bottle with a few ice cubes.

### ELECTROLYTE BEACH DRINK  *MAKES 1 QUART*

1 cup aloe juice

3 cups coconut water

Pinch of pink salt

Combine the aloe juice, coconut water, and salt in a 1-qt insulated water bottle with a few ice cubes.

### CUCUMBER LIME ALOE-ADE  *MAKES 1 QUART*

1 cup aloe juice

3 cups water

Juice of one lime

One 2-inch piece cucumber, sliced into ⅛-inch rounds

Combine the aloe juice, water, lime juice, and cucumber in a 1-qt insulated water bottle with a few ice cubes.

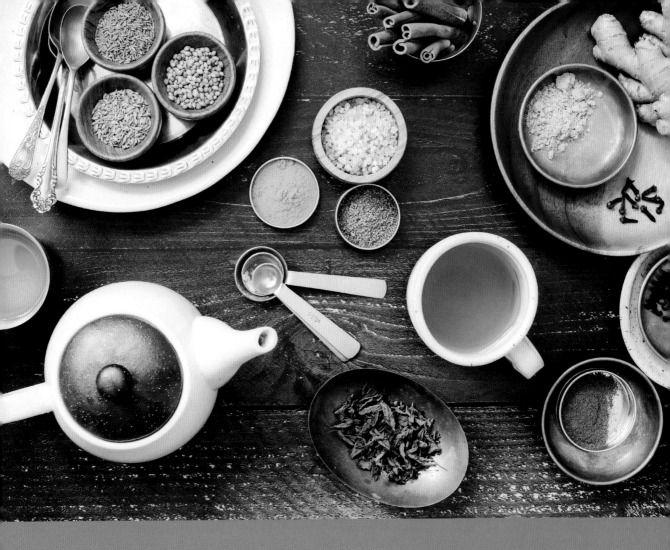

# KASHAYAMS

A kashayam is a strong tea made by boiling herbs or spices in hot water for five to twenty minutes. The longer it boils, the stronger it will be. These recipes are for hot herbal beverages to be used before, during, or after meals to improve appetite and digestion. They can also be sipped all day for purification and immunity boosting or for relief of cold symptoms such as cough and congestion.

The use of spices and herbs to support the lungs, sinuses, and digestive organs goes back as far as we can find in any culture. Sometimes suppressing symptoms with cold medicines while continuing to overwork the body can make a cold stick around longer, while one of these remedies can support your body in doing what it wants to do: move the cold out. Once this cycle is completed, you will feel full power again.

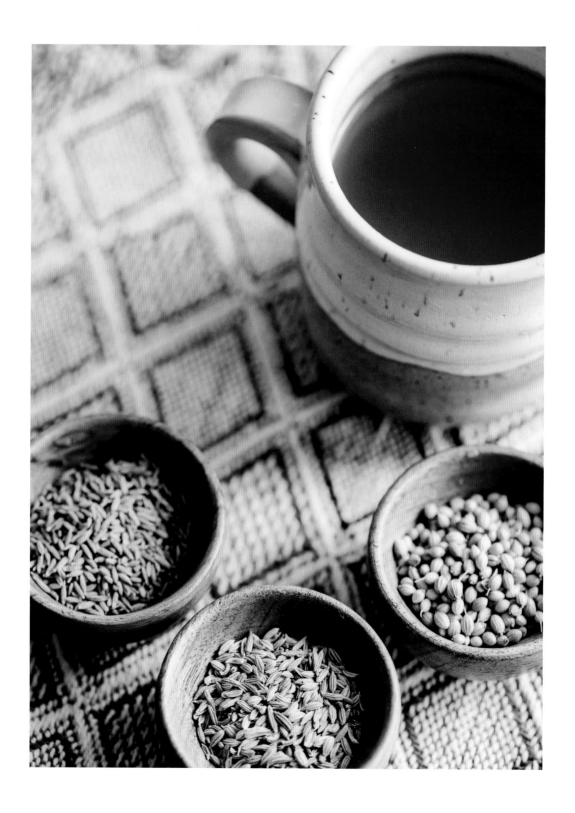

# CUMIN-CORIANDER-FENNEL TEA

*MAKES 1 QUART* This recipe, also known as "CCF Tea," is an Ayurveda panacea for gut health and blood purification. Get a minicleanse going by sipping this blend every 15–20 minutes for 1–3 days, along with a healthy diet.

| | |
|---|---|
| 1 qt water | In a medium saucepan, bring the water to a boil. |
| 1 tbsp cumin seed | Add the cumin, coriander, and fennel seeds and turn the heat down |
| 1 tbsp coriander seed | to simmer, covered, for 15 minutes. Alternatively, boil for 5 minutes, remove from heat, and leave covered to soak for 15 minutes more. |
| 1 tbsp fennel seed | Strain the liquid directly into a thermos to keep warm for the day. |

## SUMMERTIME CCF TEA

Contributor Erin Casperson, dean of Kripalu School of Ayurveda, calls CCF Tea the "Windex of Ayurveda." Here is what she says about the beloved remedy: "I have to confess, I don't like it because I taste cumin all day long. I realized I could make my own version, replacing the cumin with cardamom, and it is amazing for me. I digest it so well. It decreases my gas and bloating, and I don't burp up cumin all day." What a testimony! If you are someone who gets cumin burps, try this version. I, for one, would use it at room temperature in summer, as its spices are all cooling.

1 qt water

1 tbsp fennel seeds

1 tbsp coriander seeds

5 cardamom pods

In a medium saucepan, bring the water to a boil.

Add the fennel and coriander seeds and cardamom pods and turn the heat down to simmer, covered, for 15 minutes. Alternatively, boil for 5 minutes, remove from heat, and leave covered to soak for 15 minutes more. Strain directly into a thermos to keep warm for the day.

# TRIPHALA TEA

*MAKES 1 CUP* Triphala, a mixture of three fruits that are dried and roasted, tones each of the digestive organs—the stomach, small intestine, and large intestine. This optimizes your digestion, assimilation, and absorption of food nutrients. This nutrition then creates optimized bodily tissues. *And* triphala ensures that wastes move out of the colon. Triphala's benefits cast a wide net. It's amazing stuff!

**½ tsp triphala powder**

**1 cup hot water**

Place the triphala in the bottom of a mug.

Pour the water over the powder, cover, and steep for 10 minutes.

You can drink the sediment at the bottom of the infused water, or strain it out. Wait 2-3 hours after dinner to drink this tea.

### HOW TO USE TRIPHALA

As a general aspect of health maintenance, ½ tsp of triphala powder nightly is a safe bet. If your stools get loose, try using ¼ tsp, or switch to amalaki powder (see chapter 9). If the stools are hard or not passing, increase to as much as 1 tsp. As with any herb, if your product is old, it won't work as well and you will need to use more. I have noticed a difference in strength when using various brands, so be open to changes in your recipe.

Triphala might taste bad to you in the beginning. The taste that is lacking in your diet will stand out, bitter, sour, sweet, and so on. As your body becomes balanced, the triphala will begin to taste mild to you. Your taste buds will tell you how it's working!

Although triphala is mild, when in doubt about taking anything that may have a laxative effect, be sure to consult your health professional.

# PEPPER-HONEY FAT BURNER

*MAKES 1 CUP* While I call this recipe a fat burner, it does a whole lot more. I make this beverage often in spring, when the rains and lack of sun are persistent for days on end. The combination of cool and moist weather can challenge the agni. You might even notice a little sniffle coming on after you eat sometimes, especially after cow's milk products. This drink can be used before meals to fire up the agni, which will initiate weight loss. Drink it 20–30 minutes before a meal. When you feel the burn, go ahead and eat. In the case of a very heavy or fatty meal, like French fries or an ice cream sundae, this drink can be taken afterward. Omit the lemon if the meal contained milk or cream.

8 oz hot water

1 tsp trikatu powder or ground black pepper

¼ cup fresh lemon juice

1 tsp honey

Add the hot water to a mug or drinking cup. Stir in the trikatu and lemon juice.

Add the honey, wait 1 minute for it to soften, and stir until dissolved.

Keep a spoon handy and stir a few times while you drink, as the powder will settle at the bottom.

## HOME REMEDY NOTES

This is some spicy hot stuff and not recommended in cases of acid stomach, rashes, or hot flashes. You can reduce the ground pepper to a comfortable level. As you get accustomed to the use of trikatu, you might find that you can use a little more. For weight loss, try drinking this daily, before your largest meal of the day, for a month or two, in conjunction with other lifestyle changes. For low agni and mucus conditions, use only as needed, maybe for a few days or a week in more extreme cases. Prolonged use can be too heating.

# FIRE UP THE AGNI TEA

*MAKES 4 CUPS*   I am including this recipe because it's quick and easy to make and you probably already have the ingredients in your house. This tea can help you out during the holidays or when you feel like your appetite is flagging. It is a strong brew and not recommended for those with a tendency toward acid stomach.

1 qt water

⅛ tsp cayenne pepper

1 tsp ground ginger

1 tsp pink salt

1 tbsp maple syrup or evaporated cane juice

Juice of 2 limes

In a medium saucepan, bring the water to a boil.

Add the cayenne, ginger, salt, and syrup. Boil for 20 minutes, then remove from heat. Allow to cool a few minutes, then add the lime juice.

Drink an 8-oz cup, warm, 20–30 minutes before each meal.

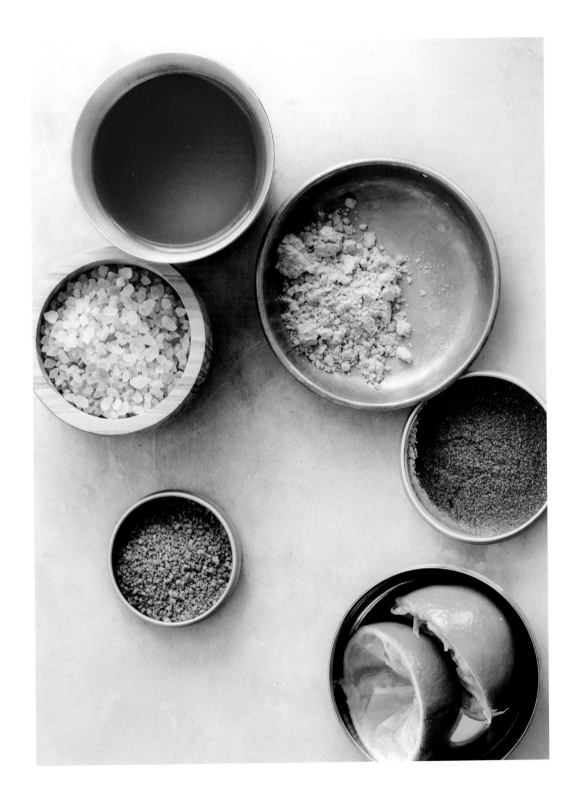

# CINNAMON SWEET-TOOTH TONIC

*SERVES 2*  Cinnamon regulates blood sugar by aiding in the breakdown of sugars. Interesting to note, this spice also creates a feeling of satiety and curbs sweet cravings. Eating a teaspoon of cinnamon every day while also eating whatever else you want may have health benefits, but using this spice to avoid overeating or "oversweeting" in the first place gives you double the effect. That's a pretty sweet deal. I recommend having this tonic as a stand-in for dessert or between meals instead of snacking.

| | |
|---|---|
| 2 cups water | In a small saucepan, bring the water to a boil, then add the cinnamon. |
| 1 tsp ground cinnamon | Cover and allow to cool for 5–10 minutes, then stir in the honey until dissolved. |
| 1 tsp raw honey | Enjoy hot or at room temperature between or after meals (like dessert!). |

# KATE'S CONGESTION REMEDY

*MAKES 4 CUPS*  This is a simple brew, but it's my go-to when I have sinus congestion or need to ward it off during cool, rainy weather. The warming and penetrating mixture of ginger and cumin dries up the mucus. Sip a cup anytime or get serious by sipping constantly throughout the day. Back off and have it only with meals if it is feeling too hot in your stomach.

| | |
|---|---|
| 1 qt water | In a medium saucepan, bring the water to a boil. |
| 1 tbsp cumin seeds | Add the cumin seeds and gingerroot, cover, and simmer for 20 minutes. |
| 2 tbsp coarsely chopped or grated fresh gingerroot | Leave the pot on the stove with the spices in it and reheat throughout the day, or strain into a thermos. |

# TALYA'S FEEL BETTER TEA

*SERVES ABOUT 4*  I asked my friend Talya Lutzker, an Ayurvedic cooking expert,[2] if she had a favorite go-to remedy. She shared her immunity-boosting cold and flu tea. Garlic is strong stuff, and while not necessary for daily use, this hot and penetrating spice is a great way to make yourself inhospitable to viral and bacterial visitors. Make and drink this tea copiously at the first sign that you are coming down with something.

12 cups water

One 2-inch piece fresh gingerroot, washed and thinly sliced

4–6 cloves garlic, minced

Juice of 1 lemon

1 tsp cayenne pepper (optional)

Raw honey, to taste

In a medium saucepan, bring the water to a boil.

Add the gingerroot and let it cook over medium-low heat for 10 minutes.

Add the garlic and cook for 5 minutes. Remove from heat.

Add the lemon juice and cayenne pepper, if using.

Once the tea has cooled a bit, serve and stir in raw honey to taste.

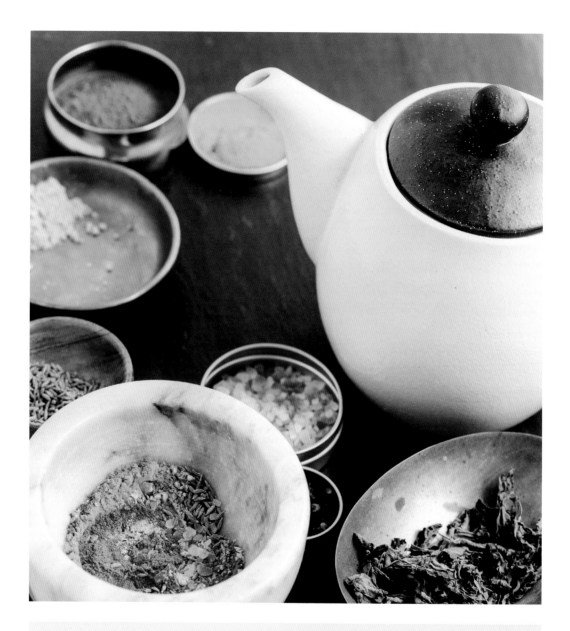

## COAT THE THROAT

If you have a speaking engagement or feel a sore throat coming on, keep a thermos of Throat Soother Tea (page 191) nearby and sip it throughout the day to ward off a cold or to support your vocal chords. I often sip this tea when I have an eight-hour teaching day.

# KASHAYAM FOR COLD CARE

*MAKES 4 CUPS*  This very strong tea covers all the bases, with eight superstar spices for cold busting. If you want to get serious about kicking that cold, this is a good bet. Make a big batch so you can sip it constantly. It is the frequency that is the key to improving your immunity and moving congestion. Put this recipe into a 1-qt thermos. Take it with you if you are going out, and sip a few ounces at least every half hour, if not more. Keep it by your bed.

1 qt water

1 tsp ground cinnamon

½ tsp ground clove

1 tsp ground ginger

1 tsp ground turmeric

¼ tsp ground black peppercorn

1 tsp cumin

¼ tsp pink salt

1 tbsp dried tulsi leaf

In a medium saucepan over high heat, bring the water to a boil.

Add the cinnamon, clove, ginger, turmeric, black pepper, cumin, salt, and tulsi. Turn the heat down to low, cover, and simmer for 20–30 minutes.

Remove from heat and transfer the tea to a thermos.

# THROAT SOOTHER TEA

*MAKES 1 QUART*  Licorice has a slippery quality, otherwise known as demulcent. Chia seeds, flaxseeds, and marshmallow root also have this action of coating the channels with moisture. In the event of a harsh, scratchy throat associated with a cough, postnasal drip, allergies, or excessive use of the voice, this tea not only soothes discomfort but also reduces inflammation and promotes healing of the mucous membranes. It is helpful for an upset stomach as well. You can find dried licorice with the bulk herbs in natural food stores.

1 qt water

1 tbsp dried licorice root or 2 tsp licorice powder

1 tsp grated fresh gingerroot

1 tsp ground turmeric

2 tsp raw honey

In a medium saucepan, bring the water to a boil.

Add the licorice, ginger, and turmeric, cover, and reduce the heat to simmer for 20 minutes.

Remove from the heat, stir in the honey, and strain through a fine sieve into a thermos.

*Note:* Licorice is not recommended for those with high blood pressure or who are using blood pressure medications. Consult your health care professional before using.

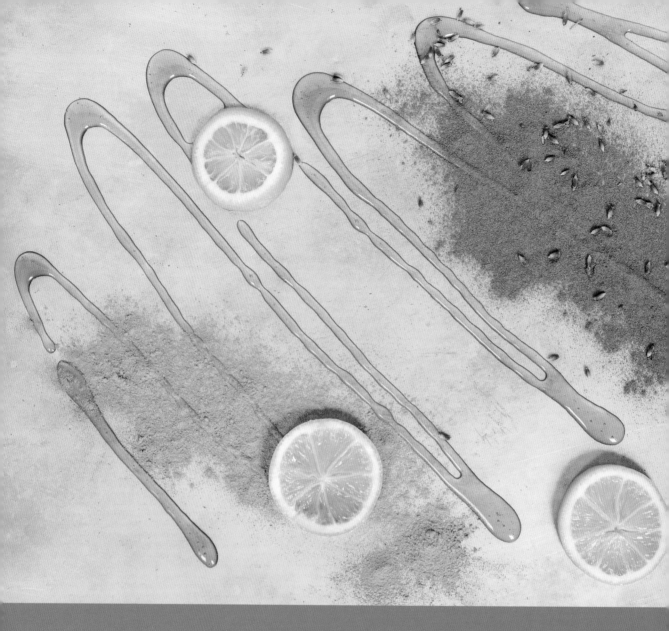

# HERBAL HONEY

Honey is used as a carrier for herbs because of its penetrating and scraping abilities. Weight-loss and cholesterol remedies often call for honey when the medicines need to make it deep into a sticky spot. Honey is also especially useful in cough and cold remedies. Thanks to its astringency, it dries up phlegm and rids the system of mucus. In this section you will find a number of honey pastes and infusion recipes that are great for coughs and colds and for burning ama.

# FREESTYLE HERBAL HONEY RECIPE

*MAKES 1 CUP*  To make an herbal honey, always begin with dried herbs, for sterility's sake. Thyme, rosemary, lavender, and tulsi are good choices. The honey must be fresh to retain its liquid state. It thickens as it ages, which makes it OK to use for pastes but too thick to infuse with dried herbs. Herbal honey is a great way to preserve and use dried herbs.

**2 tbsp dried herbs**

**8 oz fresh raw honey**

Place the herbs in the bottom of an 8-oz sterilized mason jar with a lid.

Pour the honey into the jar until it is half full, and stir to coat all of the herbs.

Top off with more honey and cover tightly.

Keep in a cool, dry place for 5–7 days. Turn it upside down every day to be sure all of the honey becomes flavored.

This will keep indefinitely.

*Note:* If you don't mind chewing on the herbs when you use the honey, either stirred into a tea or right off the spoon, it's fine to use it as is. For a clear honey infusion, strain the herbal honey through a wide mesh sieve into another sterile jar after 5–7 days.

# TULSI HONEY

*MAKES 1 CUP*  Tulsi's affinity for the circulatory system makes it a good choice for combating fevers. It also works on the respiratory system and can be useful for relieving chest colds and breathing difficulties. Mix this honey into hot water to make a tea, and drink three to four cups daily during an illness.

**2 tbsp dried tulsi**

**8 oz fresh raw honey**

Place the tulsi in the bottom of an 8-oz sterilized mason jar with a lid.

Pour the honey into the jar until it is half full, and stir to coat all of the tulsi.

Top off with more honey and cover tightly.

Strain the herbal honey through a wide mesh sieve into another sterile jar after 5–7 days.

Keep in a cool, dry place for 5–7 days. Turn it upside down every day to be sure all of the honey becomes flavored.

This will keep indefinitely.

# LAVENDER HONEY

*MAKES 1 CUP* Lavender's soothing aroma and gentle sedative effect are something I reach for in the evening as part of my get-ready-for-bed routine. Stir a teaspoon of this honey into a cup of hot water for a bedtime sleep tonic and stress reliever. Be sure to take in the aroma. For an evening sweet tooth, a taste right off the spoon is pretty special.

**2 tbsp dried lavender**

**8 oz fresh raw honey**

Place the dried lavender in the bottom of a sterilized 8-oz mason jar with a lid.

Pour the honey into the jar until it is half full, and stir to coat all of the lavender.

Top off with more honey and cover tightly.

Keep in a cool, dry place for 5–7 days. Turn it upside down every day to be sure all of the honey becomes flavored.

If you want a clear honey, strain the herbal honey through a wide mesh sieve into another sterile jar after 5–7 days.

This will keep indefinitely.

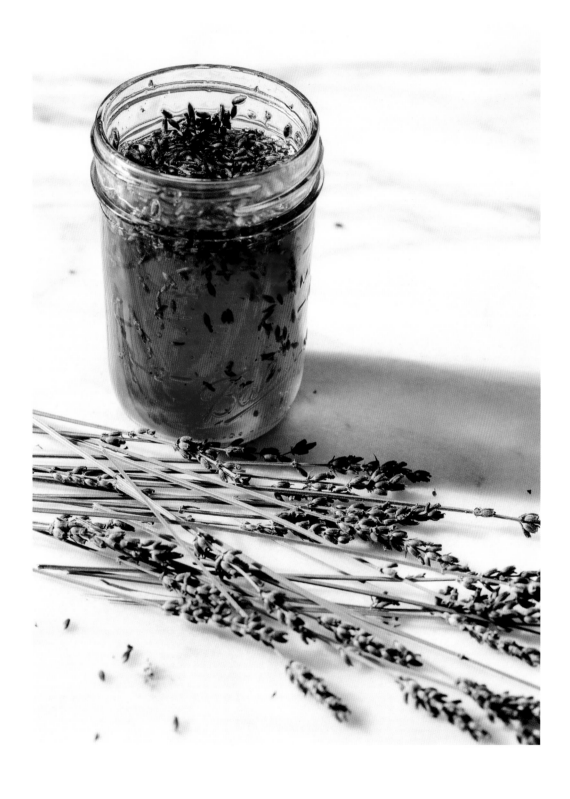

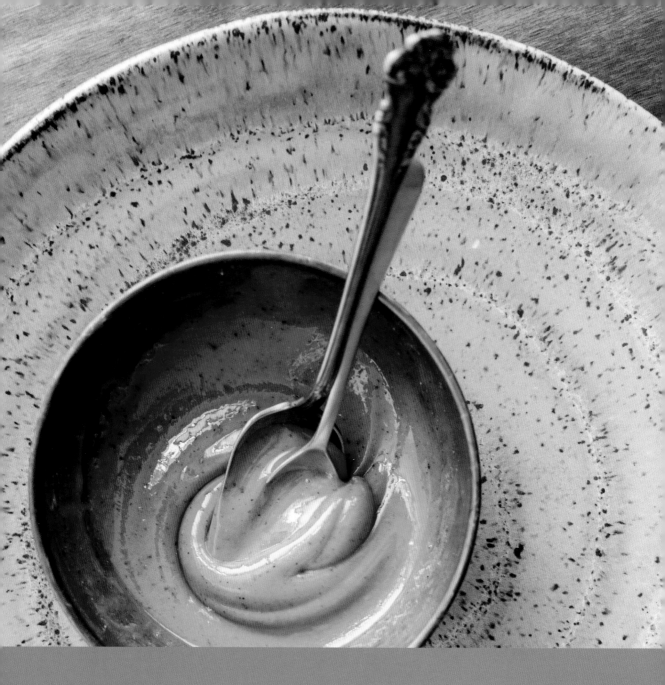

# HERBAL HONEY PASTES

Mix equal parts of powdered herbs, such as turmeric, ginger, or cinnamon, with raw honey to form a paste a little thicker than toothpaste. This can be stirred into tea or eaten off the spoon. Traditionally, bad-tasting herbs were mixed with honey, then formed into balls to be swallowed like tablets.

# TURMERIC HONEY

*MAKES ½ CUP*  This is a favorite of mine when I feel a sore throat coming on. I eat it right off the spoon and sometimes stir a teaspoon into 6 ounces of hot water a few times throughout the day to ward off a cold. I don't use a recipe but add turmeric to the honey until it reaches a paste and throw in a generous pinch of pepper. Adding pepper to turmeric remedies greatly increases its bioavailability. I make it in a bowl that sits on the counter all day to remind me to eat some. Until you get the hang of it, here is the general idea.

½ cup raw honey

1 tbsp ground turmeric

1 tsp ground black pepper

Using a sterilized 8-oz mason jar, or small glass bowl, spoon ⅔ of the honey into the jar, leaving some space for mixing. Add the turmeric and pepper, and stir until a thick paste forms.

Add the rest of the honey and stir again.

Cover and store in a cool, dark place. This will keep for a few months.

# SPICY HOT HONEY

*MAKES ½ CUP*  Clove has antibacterial as well as analgesic (pain-reducing) properties and is often used for toothaches. I love the story of the "four thieves" who robbed dead bodies during the bubonic plague without contracting the sickness by wearing clothes soaked in clove-infused vinegar over their noses and mouths. That is some serious bug defense. A hit of chili will melt and mobilize mucus to clear the nose and throat. Put this herbal honey to work when you feel early symptoms of a cold, before and after travel, anytime you have been exposed to a cold, or even when you already have one. This can be eaten off the spoon or as tea by dissolving in hot water.

½ cup raw honey

2 tsp ground ginger or 1 tbsp grated fresh gingerroot

¼ tsp ground black pepper

¼ tsp ground clove

¼ tsp cayenne pepper or red chili powder

Using a sterilized 8-oz mason jar, or small glass bowl, spoon ⅔ of the honey into the jar, leaving some space for mixing. Add the ginger, black pepper, clove, and cayenne, and stir until a thick paste forms.

Add the rest of the honey and stir again.

Cover and store in a cool, dark place. This will keep for a few months. If you used fresh ginger, keep the honey in the refrigerator and use within 2 weeks.

## GINGER NOTES

Ginger is a panacea. Its agni-boosting qualities don't create pernicious heat in the body, making it a remedy that is good for most people. The thing to know is that dried ginger is considered stronger than fresh and may cause too much heat if you already have this tendency. Fresh ginger is milder and has a sweet vipaka (aftereffect) that does not overheat the gut or the rest of the body.

# CATE STILLMAN'S BOO CANDY

*MAKES ONE 16-OUNCE JAR* When I asked my friend Cate Stillman, author of *Body Thrive* and *Master of You,* for her most-used family home remedy, she contributed this honey paste recipe. It's a spin on turmeric honey with the addition of coconut oil, which can help with absorption in the deep tissues. This is a family-size recipe. Cate and her husband take a teaspoon almost daily for healing and recovery after workouts.

2 cups ground turmeric

1 cup honey

2 tbsp coconut oil

1 tbsp ground ginger

¼ tsp ground black pepper

⅛ tsp ground cloves

Combine the turmeric, honey, coconut oil, ginger, black pepper, and cloves in a food processor and process until smooth. Mix in a large bowl with a spoon if you have no processor.

Transfer the honey to a glass jar. It keeps on the counter for up to 3 months.

---

### "BOO CANDY" FOR KIDS

Cate says, "I started keeping Boo Candy on the counter when my kid was about eighteen months old, following the doctor's recommendation not to give babies honey due to infant botulism. I'd roll the Boo Candy into pea-sized pellets to help prevent mucus, strengthen digestion, and ward off colds and flus."

# CINNAMON COUGH SYRUP

*MAKES ½ CUP*  I remember cough syrup when I was a kid. The memory of that awful taste goes along with the miserable feeling of being sick. Kids will like this one! Often coughs come on in the night and disturb sleep when sleep is just the thing you need. A quick teaspoon of this syrup can quiet the cough and get you back to bed. A teaspoon of the syrup can also be mixed into 6 ounces of water to make a soothing tea.

½ cup raw honey

2 tbsp ground cinnamon

1 tbsp fresh lemon juice

Using a sterilized 8-oz mason jar, or small glass bowl, spoon the honey into the jar, leaving some space for mixing. Add the cinnamon and lemon juice, and stir until a syrup forms.

Cover and store in the refrigerator for up to 2 weeks.

# GINGER-LEMON NECTAR

*MAKES ½ CUP*  This appetite stimulant can be used thirty minutes before meals to improve digestion. Regular use may also boost metabolism. It is so tasty I find myself having a spoonful for dessert sometimes. It also makes a very nice digestive tea when stirred into a cup of hot water after meals. Keep a jar of this on hand—I guarantee it will never go to waste because it tastes, and makes you feel, so good.

¼ cup raw honey

1 tbsp fresh lemon juice

2 tbsp grated fresh gingerroot

Spoon half of the honey into an 8-oz mason jar.

In a small bowl, mix together the lemon juice and ginger. Add to the honey.

Pour the rest of the honey into the jar and stir until uniform.

This will keep for up to 2 weeks in the refrigerator.

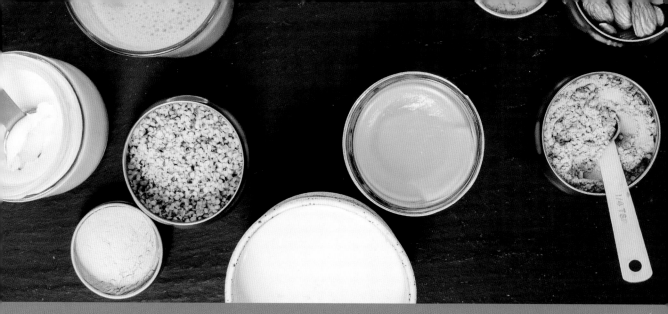

# REJUVENATING TONICS

A tonic is a medicinal substance taken to increase vigor and well-being. In Ayurveda, tonics are also known as *rasayana*, "that which nourishes the rasa dhatu." A well-nourished rasa dhatu provides nourishment for all of the other tissues. Rejuvenating tonics stave off deficiencies and provide strength. Specific combinations are revered for their abilities to increase longevity and slow the aging process. These tonics all improve sleep, brain power, and fertility.

Cow's milk is sweet, heavy, moist, cool, and oily. These qualities are all ideal for keeping the bones, nerves, and reproductive organs juicy. When these tissues dry out, we begin to see problems, such as nervous tension and infertility. Almonds and coconut are two other substances that are sweet, cooling, and oily. In the event you can't source or digest quality, grass-fed cow's milk, you can use homemade almond or coconut milk for tonics. In this section, you will find milk-based beverages with spices of both sweet and penetrating qualities, such as ginger, to help metabolize the heavy quality of the milk and assist the fats in carrying the medicinal qualities of the tonic to the deeper dhatus—the bones and marrow, the nerves (spine and brain), and the reproductive organs such as the testes, ovaries, and uterus. These deep layers are the first to become depleted, according to Ayurveda's laws of nutrition.

Nourishing tonics for the deep tissues are sometimes taken in the evening, close to bedtime, during the quiet hours when the body can use some energy to nourish the deep layers. I often recommend these recipes for a light dinner if you get home too late to eat a meal, provided you enjoyed a good breakfast and lunch that day. A rejuvenating tonic is a great way to replace what your body has lost, provide comfort and deep nourishment, and promote sound sleep.

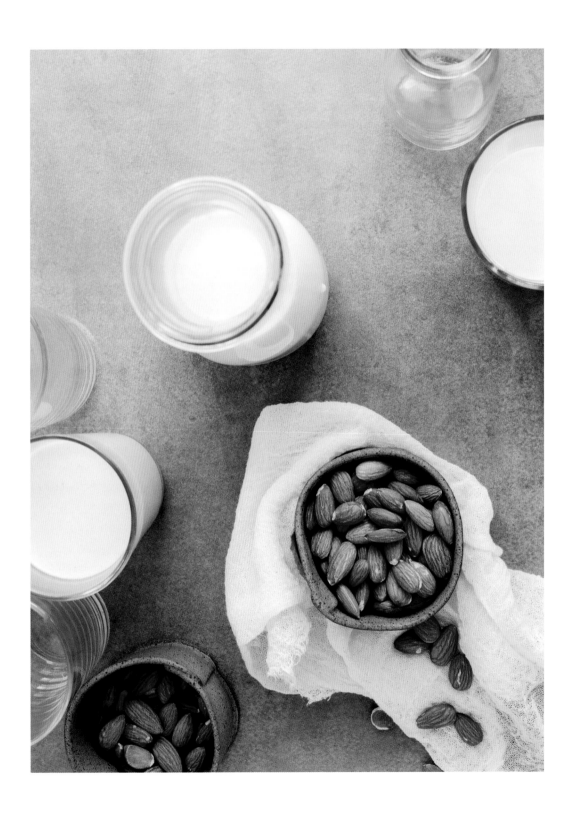

# BASIC ALMOND MILK RECIPE

*MAKES 1 QUART*  Cool, sweet, and easy to digest, homemade almond milk is good for all doshas. Most store-bought almond milks contain very little actual almonds these days. This recipe is just almonds and water, and it provides a base for many of the tonic recipes that follow.

**⅔ cup raw almonds**

**4 cups water**

Soak the almonds for at least 6 hours and up to overnight. If you oversoak, your milk will go bad faster.

Drain and rinse.

Using a hand blender or carafe blender, blend the almonds with ½ cup of the water to make a paste. Add the remaining 3½ cups of water and blend on high for 1 minute.

Strain through a fine sieve or cheesecloth into a glass container. The pulp can be used for baking and to thicken cereals and soups.

The almond milk will keep for up to 5 days in the refrigerator.

# BASIC COCONUT MILK RECIPE

*MAKES 1 QUART*  Milk made from coconut meat is especially good for pitta types due to its cooling nature. Served warm, its good fats are beneficial for vata types as well. You will find it's a lot more affordable than making almond milk. It is rich and delicious but can cause an increase in kapha because it is both cool and oily. I tend to make this one more in summer.

**4 cups water**

**1 cup unsweetened shredded coconut**

Boil 1 cup of the water and soak the coconut in it for 5 minutes. I do this right in the blender carafe.

Blend on high to make a paste, then add the remaining 3 cups of water at room temperature and blend on high for 1 minute.

Strain through a fine sieve or cheesecloth into a glass container. The pulp can be used for baking and to thicken cereals and soups.

The milk will keep for up to 5 days in the refrigerator.

# LUBRICATION STATION

*MAKES 1 CUP* This two-ingredient classic is chiefly a bedtime remedy for constipation caused by dryness. Dry quality can cause other problems too, and this combo can be used to soothe the nerves, aid sleeping and pooping after travel, and increase moisture throughout the body. You can add a touch of maple syrup to make it more delicious, if you like.

1 cup milk of choice (cow, almond, or coconut)

1 tsp ghee

Pinch of digestive spice: ground ginger, cinnamon, nutmeg, pepper, or cumin

In a small saucepan over medium heat, warm the milk, ghee, and spice to steaming.

Whisk to a uniform consistency with a fork or a milk frother.

Pour the milk into a mug and drink immediately.

### FAT IS LOVE

Fat gets a bad rap in Hollywood, but Ayurveda loves it! The word for "oil" (that which lubricates), *snehana*, also means love. Fats in the diet are responsible for beautiful, lustrous eyes and skin, and they provide a satisfied, contented feeling from the inside out.

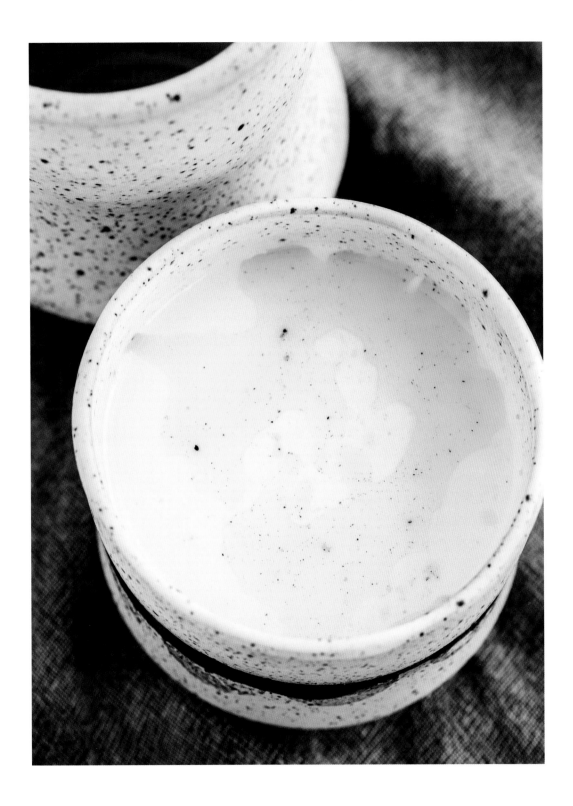

# STRESS-BE-GONE TONIC

*MAKES 1 CUP*  Ashwagandha is an adaptogenic herb, similar in qualities to South America's maca root, with an affinity for the male system, though it benefits both men and women by providing stress resistance. Sometimes stress weakens the body physically, but emotional and subtle factors can also cause stress that weakens the entire system. A tonic like ashwagandha milk is something to lean on in cold weather, during travel, and for general stress management. (Ashwagandha root does have a heating vipaka, so consult a practitioner before using it in hot weather or if you already have excessive heat.)

1 cup milk of choice (cow, almond, or coconut)

1 tsp ashwagandha powder

⅛ tsp ground nutmeg

¼ tsp ground cinnamon

¼–½ tsp ground ginger

1 tsp maple syrup (optional)

In a small saucepan, warm the milk, ashwagandha, nutmeg, cinnamon, ginger, and maple syrup, if using, until steaming. Stir with a fork, whisk, or use an electric milk frother to blend the spices into the milk.

Pour it into a mug, have a seat, and sip slowly.

## MAKE IT IN BULK

If you make this recipe a lot, measure out the herbs and spices in bulk: 1 cup ashwagandha powder, 2 tbsp ground nutmeg, ¼ cup ground cinnamon, and ¼ cup ground ginger. Combine and keep them in a glass jar for easy use.

# BONE BUILDER

*SERVES 1* This rich, sweet, and thick tonic is like a warm smoothie. The combination of milk, dates, almonds, and ashwagandha targets the deep tissue layers and brings building qualities. Asthi dhatu, the bone layer, naturally begins to break down as we age. This recipe is an anti-aging tonic that builds ojas as well as bones. I often recommend it for kids and teenagers too, especially athletic ones. Almond or coconut milk can be substituted if you can't tolerate cow's milk.

Enjoy it as a light dinner or dessert. If you need the nutrition, drink it nightly; otherwise, consider using it one to three times weekly in cold weather.

**10 almonds, soaked overnight**

**2 Medjool dates**

**1 cup cow's milk**

**2 tsp ashwagandha powder**

**1 tsp ground ginger**

**½ tsp ground cinnamon**

**⅛ tsp ground cardamom**

Drain and rinse the almonds, then remove and discard the skins.

Remove the pits from the dates. If the date pieces are not soft and moist, soak them in a few tablespoons of hot water for a few minutes.

In a medium saucepan over medium heat, warm the dates, milk, almonds, ashwagandha, ginger, cinnamon, and cardamom until steaming.

Using a hand blender, blend all the ingredients until smooth.

Transfer the drink to a mug or bowl, and have a spoon on hand!

# AYUR-EVENING TREAT

*SERVES 1* This recipe is a contribution from Cara Brostrom, our star photographer, and is a tried-and-true favorite of this working yogi mom. It is Cara's own variation on the ojas milk recipe I share with participants on my fall cleanse. After a period of cleansing, rejuvenating the deep tissues for the upcoming cold winter season is simple when it tastes like this. Almonds, dates, and digestive spices come together for an easy-to-digest sweet treat with health benefits. Beats a cookie anytime.

**1–2 pitted Medjool dates**

**8 oz almond milk**

**⅛ tsp ground cardamom**

**¼ tsp ground ginger**

**⅛ tsp ground turmeric**

Soak the dates in hot water for 15 minutes to soften, then drain. In a medium saucepan over medium heat, warm the almond milk, drained dates, cardamom, ginger, and turmeric (do not boil).

Using a hand blender, puree the mixture to desired smoothness, transfer to a thermos or mug, and drink warm—or eat with a spoon if you like it a little chunky.

This treat makes a nice dessert after a lighter meal or after a serious day.

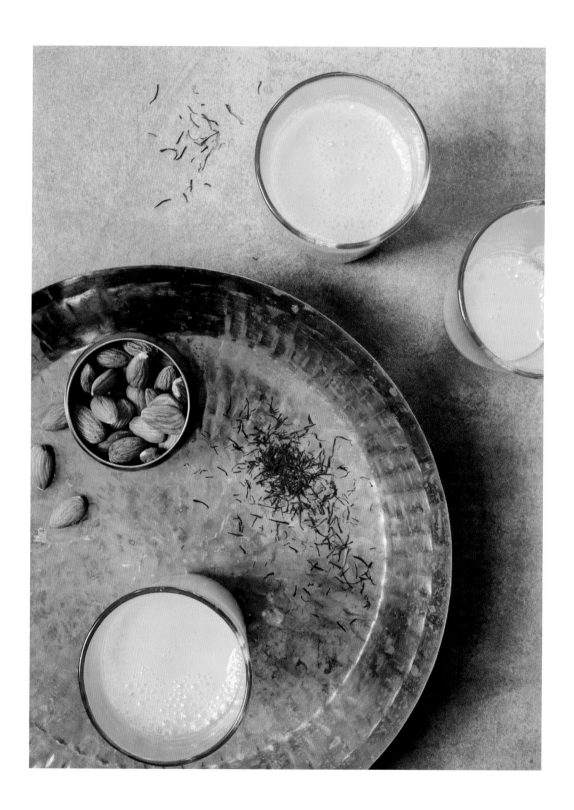

# RADIANCE SAFFRON-ALMOND MILK

*SERVES 2* Saffron and almonds are both revered as beauty tonics and are used internally as well as topically. Cleopatra added saffron to her baths, while ancient Greeks are said to have mounted perilous voyages in search of this colorful spice. Its color is like the glow of embers and fosters tejas, the subtle glow of fire element in the body and intellect. Saffron is an aphrodisiac, anti-inflammatory, free-radical busting, glow-inducing prize that is combined with almond milk to target the skin and reproductive tissues. This brightly colored, rich, and tasty recipe can also be enjoyed as a health beverage anytime. Think radiance.

¼ cup almonds, soaked overnight

2 cups water

1 pinch ground cardamom or 1 pod, cracked

1 tsp saffron threads

1 tbsp raw honey

Drain and rinse the almonds, then remove and discard the skins. They slide off easily when you pinch the almond between your pointer finger and thumb.

Using a carafe blender or a hand blender, grind the almonds with ½ cup of the water to make a smooth paste. Add the remaining 1½ cups of water, and blend.

Transfer the almond mixture to a small saucepan, and add the cardamom. Crush the saffron threads with your fingertips and add to the saucepan. Bring the mixture to steaming over medium heat.

Turn the heat down to low and simmer for 10 minutes.

Remove from the heat and stir in the honey. Pull out the cardamom pod (if using) with a teaspoon.

Pour the milk into mugs and serve warm.

# JUICY JOINTS HEMP MILK

*SERVES 1* Hemp seeds are special because they contain lubricating oils, as well as anti-inflammatory properties. Native to North America, hemp is a plant-based, often-overlooked superfood that grows easily and is a digestible source of oily quality. Overworked or older joint tissues can be painful and limit physical activity, which brings its own host of problems. Keeping the joints happy is a key aspect to healthy aging. A long time ago, I met an athlete who swore by hemp oil—she ate one tablespoon daily, and if she didn't, she said her knees would start to creak. In my experience, there's truth to that story. Remember not to boil it, as hemp oils will break down at higher than medium heat.

1 cup water

¼ cup hemp seeds

½ tsp ground turmeric

2 tsp ashwagandha

1 tsp ground ginger

Dash of ground black pepper

Dash of pink salt

1-2 tsp evaporated cane juice (optional)

In a small saucepan, heat 1 cup of the water almost to boiling. Remove from the heat and soak the hemp seeds and turmeric in it for 5 minutes.

Using a carafe blender or hand blender, grind the water with the hemp and turmeric with the ashwagandha, ginger, pepper, salt, and cane juice, if using, to a make a paste, adding more water if needed. Blend until smooth.

Drink immediately, anytime of day.

# THE JUICE ON JOINTS

There are two sources of joint pain: dryness and inflammation. Dryness breaks down joint surfaces and reduces the amount of synovial fluid in the joint itself. Pain in one joint can be structural, whereas pain in many joints belies a systemic situation. I've seen people's joint pain go away with lubrication through ghee or hemp oil, after cleansing, and with sustained dietary changes such as removing nightshade vegetables or wheat (both of which can sometimes cause inflammation).

In the event of dryness, pain will be aggravated by cold, dry weather and by ingesting cold, dry food such as raw vegetables, crackers, and ice water. Joints are likely to make cracking sounds, especially if you have a cold, dry constitution. Many of the recipes in this section will bring moisture to the body, and Juicy Joints Hemp Milk in particular targets the joints. General vata management, increasing ghee and hemp in the diet, and practicing oil massage regularly can help. Be on your game in cold weather.

Inflammation can make the joints, especially the small ones in hands and feet, feel swollen and thick. This will increase in hot or moist weather and with the intake of heating acidic foods like coffee, alcohol, and peppers. There is often a digestive component to the condition. In this case, the pain may increase after eating difficult-to-digest foods such as dairy, wheat, and fatty or fried foods.

In the Ayurvedic view, improving the agni, burning ama, and cooling the blood (see aloe cooler recipes, page 174) reduce inflammation. Do not forget: relaxing the mind cools the blood. While it's too much to go into here, stress is absolutely involved in many cases of inflammation. (Check out *Everyday Ayurveda Cooking for a Calm, Clear Mind* to investigate this avenue.)

Systemic situations can be complicated, and while I share these general principles to shine some light on sources of joint pain, it's a good idea to seek out a professional about anything chronic.

# TURMERIC MILK MACCHIATO

*SERVES 1*  If you think of my usual turmeric milk recipe as a latte, this is more of a macchiato. Stronger medicine, smaller volume. Sometimes I drink it down like a shot rather than sipping. I find that less liquid digests easier after having eaten. In the morning, I go latte style and add a little sweetener. This tonic is well known in the yoga and Ayurveda traditions for a long list of benefits, namely as an anti-inflammatory, bone nourisher, and immunity booster. The synergistic combination of turmeric, coconut, ginger, and pepper nourishes as well as heals deep tissue cells.

½ cup milk of choice (whole cow's, almond, or coconut)

1 tsp ground turmeric

½ tsp ground ginger

1 tsp coconut oil

Pinch of ground black pepper

Honey, for serving (optional)

In a small saucepan over medium-high heat, combine the milk, turmeric, ginger, coconut oil, and pepper and heat, uncovered, for 2–4 minutes, or until steaming.

Remove from the heat and whisk by hand or with an electric milk frother until combined.

Pour the drink into a mug, sweeten with honey, if using, and drink immediately.

---

### MEET DAD WHERE HE'S AT

I've been trying to get my dad into turmeric milk for a while. Finally, he told me he was trying it, but it wasn't coming out very well. Turns out he was doing a vigilante twist on my recipe—making it in the microwave. The coconut oil sat like an oil slick, and the spices clumped up. Now, I understand Dad wants to do the whole thing right in the glass measuring cup and cut out the dishwashing. I get it. So, although the microwave might not be ideal, I'm still happy he's on the nightly self-care bandwagon. I bought him an electric milk frother to stick in the cup after heating, and the final product is now a beloved treat!

It's easy to talk ourselves out of self-care by saying, "Nah, it's too many dishes to cook it, and I know I'm not supposed to microwave it." The desire to spend a doable amount of time doing something beneficial for yourself is the goal. It's not about preparing it perfectly; it's about doing it at all. So, give yourself a break, choose your battles, and make it work for you. Once you get the party started, things will continue to evolve. Next time I visit, maybe Dad will be making ghee in the microwave.

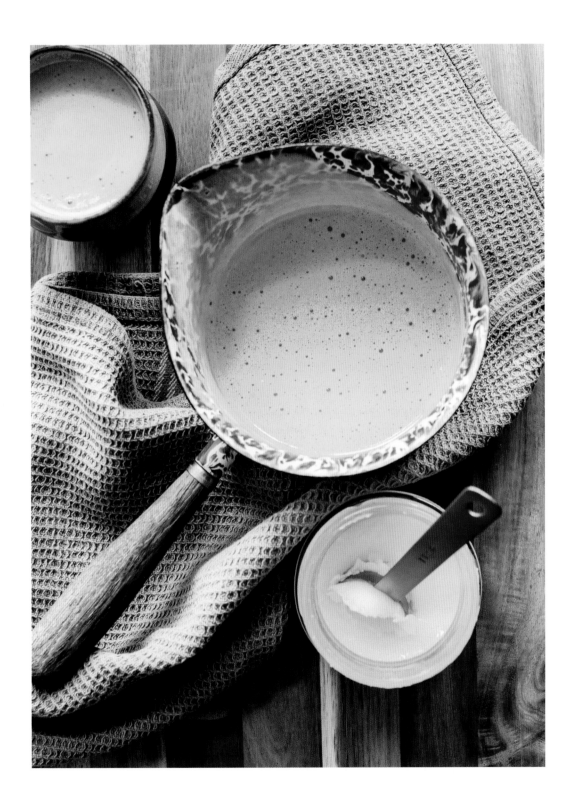

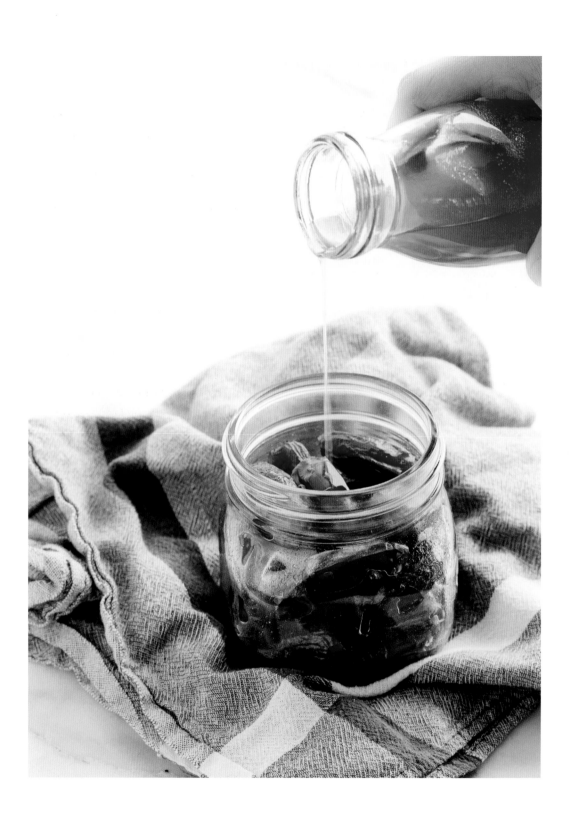

# JAR O' OJAS (SPICED DATES IN GHEE)

*MAKES 16 OUNCES*   A prized aphrodisiac, the date when ghee-soaked and spiced is a rasayana love potion. Beyond increasing libido, this combination builds ojas and promotes formation of the deepest bodily tissues. It is often used in cases of debility and lack of energy, as well as when unwanted weight loss has occurred. It's a heavy mix, and the spices are key to digesting it. If you have ama or weak agni, do not use this recipe. If you have strong agni, a date a day is a super rebuilding food after cleansing, competitive sports, or weight loss due to illness. Do not sit down with the jar; you won't stop at just one!

2 pinches saffron thread

¼ tsp ground cinnamon

¼ tsp ground cardamom

¼ tsp ground ginger

1 cup ghee, or enough to cover

1½ cups pitted deglet noor dates, cut in half

Using a mortar and pestle, grind the saffron to a fine powder. Add the cinnamon, cardamom, and ginger, and grind together.

In a medium saucepan over low heat, warm the ghee until liquid, and add the spice mixture.

Pack the dates tightly into a 16-oz mason jar with a lid. Make sure the jar is absolutely clean and dry.

Pour the spiced ghee over the dates. Cover tightly and shake well.

Let the dates soak for 1 day before enjoying. These will keep at room temperature for up to 3 months.

*Note:* Dried dates work better than moist Medjool dates. Deglet noor may be the easiest for you to find, but if you have access to other varieties of dried dates, those will work too. You may have to soak very dry dates longer to soften them.

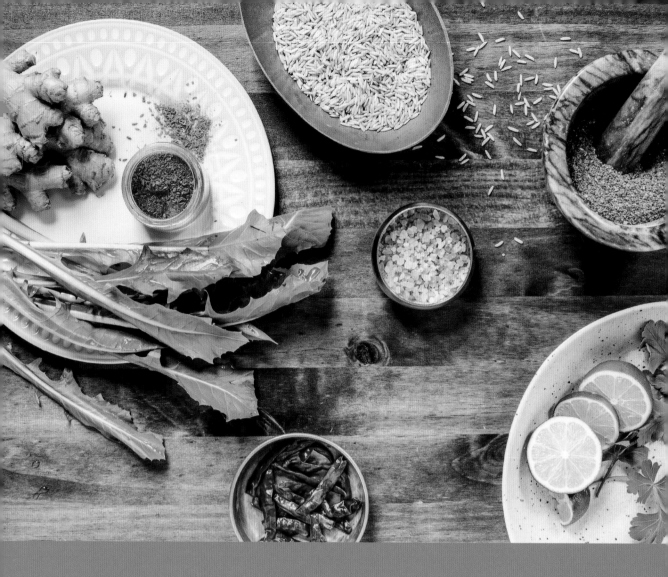

# MEDICINAL SOUPS AND MORE

There is a reason grandmas all over the world make you soup when you are sick. I'm sure you've experienced a time when soup was a craving that helped you get well, whether it's America's chicken noodle soup, veggie broth, or India's rasam. Soups hydrate the body during fever or dysentery, and they are easy to digest.

   The theme here is to boost agni. It is the body's fire that burns out bugs, melts mucus, clears stagnation, and provides vitality and luster. These soups and spices include combinations that will provide nourishment without taxing the gut, and will even increase digestive power. It's no secret that food is considered medicine in Ayurveda, so please enjoy these home remedies in the form of food.

# MUCUS-BUSTING KANJEE

*SERVES 4-6*   Barley, in combination with ginger and cumin, has the ability to remove excess moisture. This soup helps in heating and drying up excess mucus, such as when you have a stuffy or runny nose or allergies. Try this for breakfast, or fast on it for a day to bust up lingering congestion.

1 cup barley, soaked overnight and strained

10 cups water

¼ tsp salt

1 tsp ground cumin

1 tsp ground turmeric

1 tsp ground ginger

½ tsp ground black pepper

In a large pot over low heat, boil the barley, water, salt, cumin, turmeric, ginger, and pepper together, partially covered, for 1 hour or until the grain breaks up and the soup appears creamy.

Stir well and ladle into soup bowls.

Serve the soup warm as a light meal, or throughout the day to hydrate and nourish when fasting. Add more hot water to desired consistency.

# HEALING KANJEE

*SERVES 4*  Kanjee ("KAHN-jee") is a very simple food that provides nourishment and hydration without overworking the digestion. It goes well with resting and recuperating. Traditionally, and to this day, in Ayurveda clinics and hospitals, the digestion is nursed back to health with grain soup of increasing thickness as the patient begins to feel better. You can use this food when you don't have an appetite for much, after a stomach bug, or during the flu.

1 cup brown basmati rice

10 cups water

¼ tsp salt

¼ tsp ground cumin

¼ tsp ground turmeric

¼ tsp ground ginger

*Note*: Replace the cumin with 1 tsp cinnamon, if you want a sweet version

In a large pot over low heat, boil the rice, water, salt, cumin, turmeric, and ginger together, partially covered, for 1 hour or until the rice breaks up and the soup appears creamy.

Stir well and ladle into soup bowls.

Serve kanjee warm as a light meal, or throughout the day to hydrate and nourish when fasting.

*Note:* If your gut is up to the task and you want more food, begin to add 1 cup of chopped carrot or ¼ cup chopped dates or raisins to the mix.

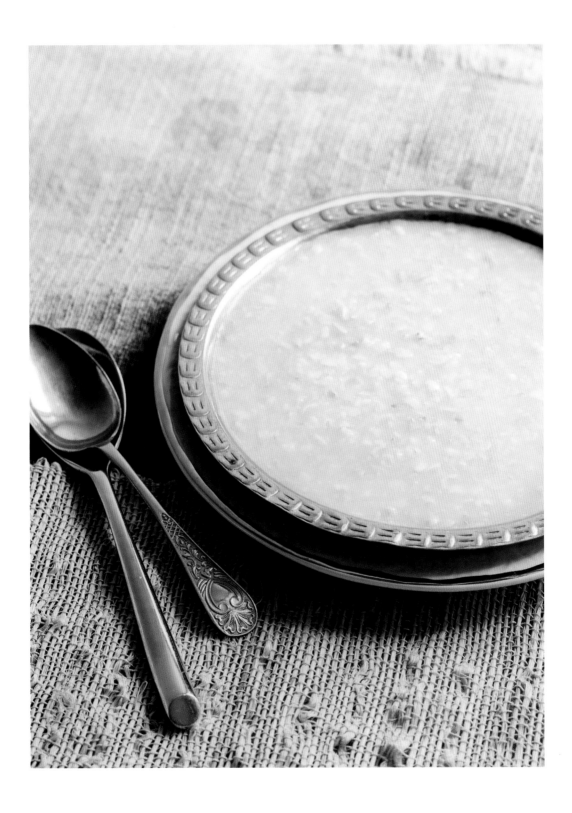

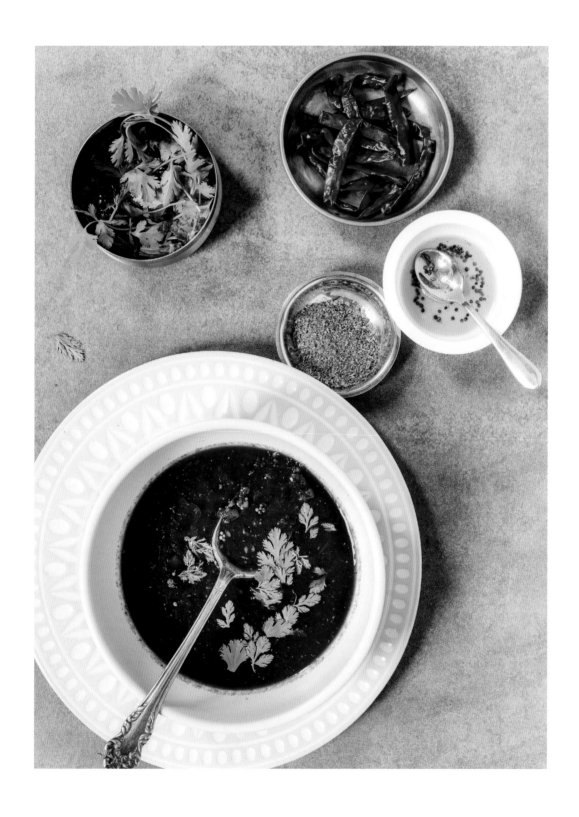

# PEPPER RASAM

*SERVES 2*   In India if you have a cold, someone is going to offer you rasam. This spicy, tomato-based soup is the "chicken noodle soup" of India for common colds. It is a serious melt-your-mucus recipe with red chili and peppercorn. Rasam is also served as a starter to improve the digestive fire before a big meal. If you are feeling blocked due to a cold, however, try sipping a cup of this brothlike soup to ease congestion. Have some tissues ready!

**SPICE MIXTURE**

2 dried red chilies

2 tbsp coriander seed

1 tbsp black peppercorn

½ tbsp cumin seed

**SOUP**

2 ripe tomatoes, chopped (plum variety)

1 tbsp tamarind paste (see note below)

Pinch of hing

¼ tsp ground turmeric

¼ tsp salt

½ cup water

**TEMPERING**

2 tsp ghee

¼ tsp mustard seed

1–2 tbsp chopped cilantro, for garnish

In a pan, dry roast the chilies, coriander, black pepper, and cumin until fragrant, just a few minutes. Cool the mixture, then grind to a powder in a coffee or spice grinder.

In a medium saucepan over medium-high heat, bring the tomatoes, tamarind, hing, turmeric, and salt to a boil. Reduce the heat and add the spice mixture and water. Simmer, partially covered, for 20 minutes.

In a small saucepan over medium heat, warm the ghee. Add the mustard seeds and cover while they pop, about 1 minute. Remove from heat.

Add the ghee and mustard mixture to the rasam and stir.

Serve the rasam in bowls and garnish with the cilantro.

*Note:* Though I highly recommend using the tamarind paste, if you can't find it, replace it with 1 tbsp lime juice or apple cider vinegar.

# DR. CLAUDIA'S AGNI SOUP

*SERVES 2-4*  When I asked Dr. Claudia Welch, a doctor of Chinese medicine as well as an Ayurvedic practitioner, if she had a favorite home remedy, she offered this miso soup recipe. Miso soup is like kanjee or rasam—it's a mainstay. You can make a simple savory broth by adding miso to hot water. This soup will have more of a Chinese flavor, due to the soy sauce, seaweed, and vinegar. It's a great meal after being out in the cold.

3-4 tbsp sunflower or safflower oil

1 tbsp toasted sesame oil

1 onion, diced small

2 medium carrots, grated

½ cup celery, thinly sliced

½ medium daikon, grated (optional)

2-3 tbsp finely grated fresh gingerroot

½ tsp ground black pepper

½ cup dulse seaweed, rinsed

4 cups water, plus additional if needed

1 tbsp kudzu

1 large handful thin rice noodles

2-3 tbsp rice vinegar

2 tbsp maple syrup

2-3 tbsp soy sauce

1 bunch scallions, finely chopped

1-2 tbsp red miso

In a large pot or sauce pan over medium heat, heat the sunflower and sesame oils. Add the onions and sauté until they're translucent, about ten minutes. Add the carrots and celery, and sauté another minute. Add the daikon, and sauté another minute.

Add the ginger, black pepper, seaweed, and 2 cups of the water. Simmer 10 minutes.

Add the remaining 2 cups of water, plus more if needed to cover the vegetables. In the meantime, in a small bowl dissolve the kudzu in a few tablespoons of cold water. Bring the soup to a boil, and add the noodles, rice vinegar, kudzu, maple syrup, and soy sauce, and cook until the noodles are tender, 3-5 minutes.

Turn off the heat and add the scallions and miso (the miso should not be boiled).

Ladle the soup into bowls and serve.

# ROASTED EGGPLANT SOUP

*SERVES 2*  Eggplant is among a group of foods that encourage downward movement in the body, which is called *anulomina*. Eating eggplant can be helpful in constipation, for irregular or scanty periods, and even for relieving congestion by clearing the digestive channels and making some room for movement. Here I have kept the eggplant at the forefront and mixed in some agni-boosting herbs and the lubrication of ghee, but if you have another version you like, maybe with lots of garden herbs, that will work too!

2 tbsp ghee

2 medium eggplants

1 small red onion, chopped

2 large celery sticks, chopped

⅛ tsp hing powder

1 tsp ground cumin

1 tsp ground coriander

2 cups vegetable broth

½ tsp pink salt (omit if your broth is salted)

Ground black pepper, fresh parsley, or thyme, to garnish

Preheat oven to 400 degrees.

Rub ¼ tsp of the ghee onto the skin of the eggplants and place them on a baking dish.

Bake until the eggplants collapse, 45–50 minutes. Allow them to cool enough to handle.

Scoop the eggplant flesh from the skin into a mixing bowl. Discard the skin.

In a large saucepan over medium heat, warm the remaining ghee. Add the onion and celery, and sauté until soft.

Add the hing, cumin, and coriander, and stir.

Add the eggplant and broth (and salt, if using), stir, and turn the heat down to simmer. Cook, covered, for 20 minutes.

Using an immersion blender, puree the soup until smooth.

Ladle into soup bowls, and top with pepper and fresh herbs to serve.

*Note:* Try using one of my spice mixes instead of the cumin and coriander.

# SPICY DANDELION GREEN SOUP

*SERVES 2*  In spring, take advantage of the blood-cleansing powers of fresh dandelion. After a long winter, the digestive and circulatory systems need to break up the heavy and dense qualities accumulated to stay warm and moist. This soup is a great way to support the process, and an excellent addition to a spring cleanse. Keep your eyes peeled for the dandelion greens to show up—they are only around for a short while. When you can get them, try having this soup daily for a few days.

One 3-inch piece gingerroot, peeled and coarsely chopped

1 tsp Cumin Coriander Fennel Turmeric powder (see page 231)

⅛ tsp hing

¼ tsp ground black pepper

½ tsp pink salt

Pinch of red chili powder or cayenne pepper (optional)

2 cups vegetable broth

2 cups chopped Swiss chard

1 cup chopped dandelion leaves

1 cup chopped parsley

In a soup pot over low/medium heat, dry roast the ginger, CCFT powder, hing, black pepper, salt, and chili powder, if using, for 20–30 seconds, until fragrant.

Add the broth to the pot, turn the heat to high, and bring to a boil. Lower heat to simmer and add the Swiss chard, dandelion leaves, and parsley.

Cook for 10 minutes, until greens are wilted and have a nice dark green color.

Using a blender or hand blender, puree the mixture until smooth. Ladle into soup bowls and serve.

*Note:* Ch-ch-changes. For more information on seasonal changes and cleanses, see chapter 6. For a green soup recipe with some protein, try Sprouted Greens Soup from *Everyday Ayurveda Cooking for a Calm, Clear Mind.* Don't forget to add some dandelion.

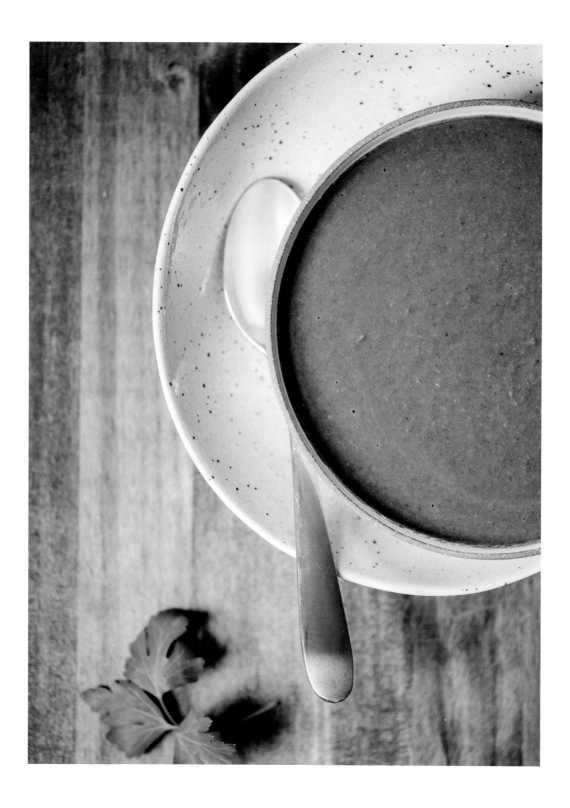

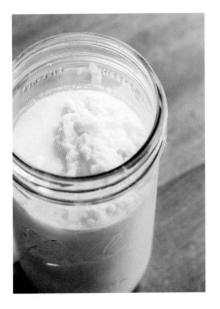

If you have my other books, you will be familiar with my lassi recipe, a drink of spiced yogurt diluted with water (not like restaurant mango lassi). You will also already know that "buttermilk" in this case is not like what goes into pancakes! For purposes of healing the digestive tract and doing deepana and pachana, the recipe for Indian buttermilk, or takra, is very specific.

Takra is the unlikely number-one digestive remedy. While its initial taste is sour, it has none of the heating qualities of a sour food. This prabhava, a special and unexplainable healing effect, makes this drink among the best substances for deepana and pachana, because it improves agni *and* digests ama. Its superpower lies in its ability to improve agni and remove excess air element from the digestive tract, thereby restoring optimal digestion and absorption of food. I have included some tips on how to use it (see page 228) and how variations on the recipe create targeted healing effects.

## TRADITIONAL TAKRA (INDIAN BUTTERMILK) *MAKES 30 OUNCES*

3 cups water (at room temperature)

¾ cup organic, natural (no thickeners added), grass-fed, whole milk yogurt

1 tsp ground ginger

⅛ tsp hing powder

1 tsp ground cumin

Pinch of pink salt

Put the water in a blender carafe, and add the yogurt.

Blend the mixture on high speed for 1 minute, until a thick foam forms on top. This is the milk solids.

Skim off the solids with a spoon and discard, or save in a glass container in the freezer until you get enough to make ghee. Repeat until there are no more fats to remove.

Add the ginger, hing, cumin, and salt, and blend for a few seconds.

Drink whenever and however you need (see How to Drink Takra, page 228). Takra does not need to be refrigerated and should not be taken cold. Make fresh daily.

*Note:* If one of the spices in this recipe bothers you, omit it. To make it pretty, add a few chopped cilantro leaves.

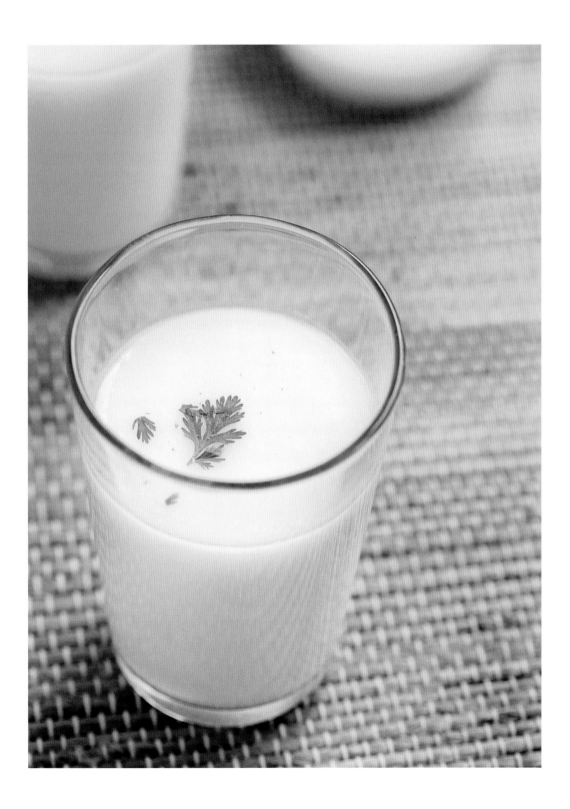

## TAKRA FOR A PICKIER PALETTE

Some people find the slightly sour, spicy, salty experience of takra off-putting, while others love it. The best remedy is the one you actually use, so here is a lighter-weight version. Replace recipe spices with any of the following:

1 tsp ground cinnamon

1 tsp ground ginger

Pinch of pink salt

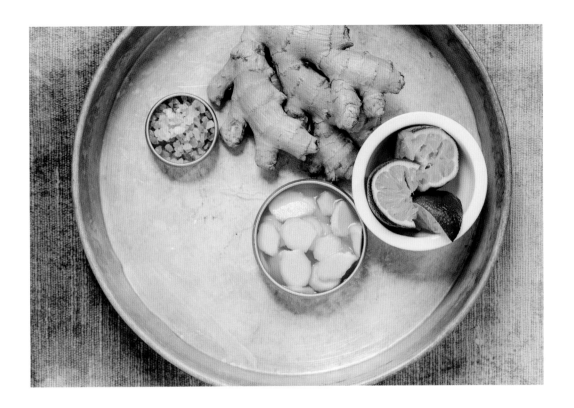

## APPETITE-BOOSTING GINGER PICKLE

*MAKES ¼ CUP* One of my besties, Erin Casperson, dean of the Kripalu School of Ayurveda, volunteered this pickle recipe as one of her favorite digestive helpers. Like all of my quick-pickle recipes, this only takes a few minutes to make and offers some real digestive power before a heavy or complicated meal and can even be taken after an indulgent meal. Don't eat this pickle if you have acid stomach.

¼ cup peeled and sliced gingerroot (⅛-inch slices)

2 tbsp fresh lime juice

⅛–¼ tsp pink salt

Place the ginger in a small jar with a lid and add the lime juice and pink salt. Cover and shake a few times, and let stand for 1 hour before eating.

Eat 1–2 slices 30 minutes before each meal to stoke digestive fire, or after a large meal to boost digestion. This pickle will keep on the counter for a few days or in the refrigerator for 7–10 days.

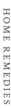

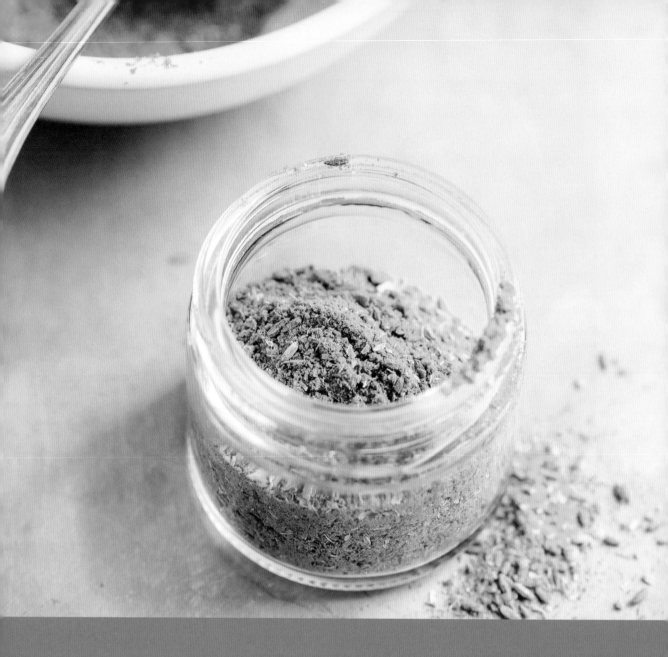

# SPICE BLENDS FOR DIGESTIVE HEALTH

These spice mixes contain culinary spices common in Ayurvedic cooking. Spices contain concentrated amounts of the six tastes and are used to bring balance to meals. For even more therapeutic effects, spices can be used before and after meals to improve appetite and digestion, as well as settle an upset stomach.

# CUMIN CORIANDER FENNEL TURMERIC MIX

*MAKES ¼ CUP*  A blend of cumin, coriander, fennel, and turmeric is a basic, often-used combination in Ayurvedic cooking. (The same mixture without the turmeric—CCF—is also commonly used.) Each of the spices has a targeted action to improve digestion, absorption, and assimilation. This mix can also be used to make a tea to be sipped throughout the day for detoxification and digestion and to promote clear skin.

1 tbsp whole
coriander seed

1 tbsp whole
cumin seed

2 tsp whole fennel
seed

1 tbsp ground
turmeric

In a heavy-bottomed pan on medium-low heat, dry roast the coriander, cumin, and fennel seeds until fragrant, a few minutes.

Transfer the seeds from the pan to a wide bowl and cool completely.

In a spice grinder or using a mortar and pestle, grind the roasted seeds to a uniform consistency.

Transfer the mixture to a bowl and stir in the ground turmeric.

Store in a small glass jar with an airtight lid.

# GINGER BLASTER

*SERVES 2*  I often use this recipe for a few days during seasonal cleanses to boost the agni. I enjoy doctoring up the ginger and think of the slices as little pizzas. The ginger's fibers give you something to chew on, and the flavors mix together in your mouth to get the appetite going. Gingerroot with smaller fingers will be tender, while big ones can be tough. It's OK to spit out the fibers after chewing. Be careful though—the taste sensation can be addictive. It is best not to continue eating these every day for more than a week or two.

One 1-inch piece
gingerroot (about
1 inch wide)

1 lemon slice

Pinch of pink salt

Peel the ginger and slice off the rough end.

Cut four coins about ⅛-inch thick. If the gingerroot is very small, like the radius of a dime, make them a little thicker.

Squeeze the lemon slice over the pieces, then sprinkle with the salt.

Eat two slices 20 minutes before meals. Wait for the appetite to increase before eating. Save the other two for your next meal; they will keep in the fridge for up to 1 week.

# COOL YOUR GUTS

*MAKES ABOUT ¼ CUP*  With all this talk of boosting agni, what about when it's too high? This spice mix settles a stomach upset by spicy food, nervousness, too much coffee, or difficult-to-digest food combinations. It is a convenient one to keep in a small container in your travel bag if you often suffer from indigestion.

1 tbsp coriander seed

1 tbsp fennel seed

¼ tsp ground cardamom or seeds of 2 green cardamom pods

1 tsp licorice powder

1 tsp evaporated cane juice

In a heavy-bottomed pan on medium-low heat, dry roast the coriander and fennel seeds until fragrant, a few minutes.

Transfer the seeds from the pan to a wide bowl and cool completely.

In a spice grinder or using a mortar and pestle, grind the roasted seeds to a uniform consistency. Add the cardamom and licorice, and grind until uniform.

In a small glass jar with an airtight lid, add the cane juice and ground spice mixture. Shake to combine.

Store in the same small glass jar.

Take 1–2 heaping tsp with a few ounces of warm water after meals or as needed.

*Note:* If you can't find licorice powder, you can make and use this blend without it.

# AFTER-MEAL CHEWING SPICE MIX

*MAKES ¼ CUP*  *The Everyday Ayurveda Guide to Self-Care* photographer, Cara Brostrom, named this mix as her most-loved digestive. After all her recipe testing and shooting, she has a lot to choose from, so this must be good! Chewing this mix postmeal will increase feelings of satisfaction, reduce dessert cravings, and settle gas and acidity in the stomach.

1 tbsp fennel seeds

1 tsp sesame seeds

2 tsp shredded coconut

Generous pinch of pink salt

In a small frying pan over low heat, dry roast the fennel seeds, sesame seeds, coconut, and salt, stirring frequently, for 2–3 minutes. Roast until fragrant, but do not burn. Transfer to a dish to cool.

Store in a small tin or jar and chew a spoonful after meals.

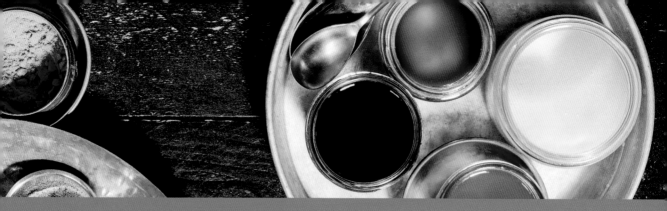

# GHRITA (HERBAL GHEE)

Ghrita is a specific group of medicines in which herbs are infused into ghee. This combination is considered special because infused ghee carries the qualities of the medicines cooked into it rather than its own qualities, which is a unique ability. The traditional making of medicinal ghee is quite a science, as is all Ayurvedic pharmacology. What you will find in this section is a slightly simplified method of infusing ghee with a few different herbs whose effects are exalted when processed in this manner. The efficacy of ghritas when traditionally prepared and used by Ayurvedic doctors is quite significant but a little beyond the DIY scope. For general purposes, periodic use of an herbal ghee to rejuvenate and provide support to specific tissue layers can be a valuable part of a longevity regimen, as long as your digestion is strong enough to break down and absorb it.

Ghee has an affinity for the deep tissue layers, especially the majja dhatu, the nerves, the brain, and the spinal cord. A few common ghritas found here are ashwagandha ghee for vitality, immunity, and male fertility; shatavari ghee for female fertility and reproductive health; and brahmi ghee for stress reduction, cognitive function, and memory.

Because ghee can be a little heavy to digest, these ghritas are often taken with a hot beverage; even just hot water will help break it down, though milk or a milk substitute may be more palatable. Enjoy ghrita daily or a few times per week, in the rejuvenating tonic recipes, or simply stirred into a warm, spiced milk of your choice. If you like the taste of ghee, you can just eat a spoonful. Make one 16-oz batch and use it until it's gone (one to three months); consider following this regimen once or twice each year, ideally as part of a seasonal cleanse.

Spiced ghee is a palatable and digestible way to get ghee into your diet, for bestowing its "one thousand good effects," including being "the best for retaining youth."[3] These digestive spiced ghee recipes metabolize easily to ensure you get the most out of your good fats—instead of just getting fat. If you have a heavier constitution, enjoy them sparingly, perhaps 1 tsp daily; a dry, undernourished body can use up to a few tablespoons daily. Spiced ghee is a delicious addition to the diet in hot cereal, on toast, added to soups, and so on.

## *Vegan Ghee*

I know some of you are wondering what to do if you're vegan. If you are not vegan, but lactose intolerant, give ghee a try because the lactose is removed through the cooking process, and I haven't yet seen anyone have difficulty digesting it. Coconut oil is the first-choice substitute, and you can certainly follow the recipes and make spiced coconut oil and herbal coconut oils. You will surely get some similar benefits by infusing herbs and spices into coconut fat. It will not have the unique and somewhat mystical properties of ghee, but I wouldn't let that stop you from making these recipes. I often refer to ghee's "golden goodness" and I do believe there is something to the color. So no one is excluded, I offer you, my friends, a vegan ghee recipe.

**MAKES 16 OUNCES**

**One 16-oz jar high-quality coconut oil**
**¼ tsp ground turmeric**
**⅛ tsp finely ground pink salt**

In a medium saucepan over medium heat, melt the coconut oil, and stir in the turmeric and salt. Simmer for 5 minutes, stirring throughout, then cool completely and pour into a sterilized glass jar. Vegan Ghee keeps at room temperature indefinitely.

**HOW TO MAKE HERBAL AND SPICED GHEE.** Herbal ghee is a two-part process, while spiced ghee is very simple. To make spiced ghee, ghee is simmered along with the powdered spices, then it is cooled and stored. To infuse herbs into ghee, first the water-soluble factors in the herb are extracted by making a decoction. This is like a very strong tea. The herb is strained out of the decoction, then the liquid is simmered along with the ghee until all of the water has evaporated. This leaves the herb and the ghee.

Some medicinal ghee takes many days to make, where aging is a part of the medicine's efficacy, and ingredients may be added at different points throughout processing. While any of these recipes can be made in an afternoon, be prepared to spend a few hours checking in on the stovetop while the decoction and then the ghee are simmering. It is important that you take the time to evaporate all the moisture out of the ghee or it can spoil.

In the event you don't see yourself brewing up these recipes at home, herbal and spiced ghees are available ready-made. Please visit the Resources section for suppliers.

## BASIC GHEE RECIPE

*MAKES ABOUT 12 OUNCES*  Think of ghee as a carrier that brings the goods, of a medicinal quality, deep into the body. Best-quality, organic butter must be the base. Ghee making is a very satisfying and fun job that turns you into a kitchen healer.

**1 lb (4 sticks) unsalted organic butter**

In a saucepan over medium heat, melt the butter.

Reduce the heat to medium-low.

After 5–10 minutes, a white froth will begin to form on the butter's surface and will create popping sounds as the moisture evaporates from the butter.

Continue to monitor; do not walk away or multitask. Notice when the popping sounds become more intermittent, then it's time to hover.

After 10–15 more minutes, when the solids begin to turn golden brown at the bottom of the pan, take it off the heat.

Cool for about 15 minutes until just warm.

Pour the butter through a strainer or cheesecloth into a clean, sterilized glass jar with a lid.

Strain off any skim of foam that might remain.

Ghee will keep, unrefrigerated, for 1–3 months. Always keep the lid on and always use a clean utensil when using or eating ghee from the jar.

*Note:* I like to make ghee with cultured butter, which is lighter and easier to digest. You will find it in your grocery store. Never compromise on the quality of butter you start with, as this is a medicine that will move deep into your body.

# GOLDEN CHAI-SPICED GHEE

*MAKES 12 OUNCES*  Infusing ghee with turmeric and chai spice brings it to another level. The qualities of the spices will increase digestibility, plus you are more likely to use this ghee in your diet because it so tasty. Try a spoonful smeared on toast, melted on a baked sweet potato, or in a hot milk. You can make a rejuvenating tonic in 2 minutes with this ghee.

12 oz ghee

2 tbsp ground ginger

2 tsp ground cardamom

1 tsp ground turmeric

In a heavy-bottomed pan over medium-low heat, melt the ghee.

Add the ginger, cardamom, and turmeric, stir, and simmer until the mixture sizzles. Continue to sauté for 2 minutes, until fragrant. Remove from the heat and let cool.

Strain the ghee through a triple layer of cheesecloth to remove the powders into a clean, sterilized glass jar with a lid, and you will be left with a golden, spiced ghee.

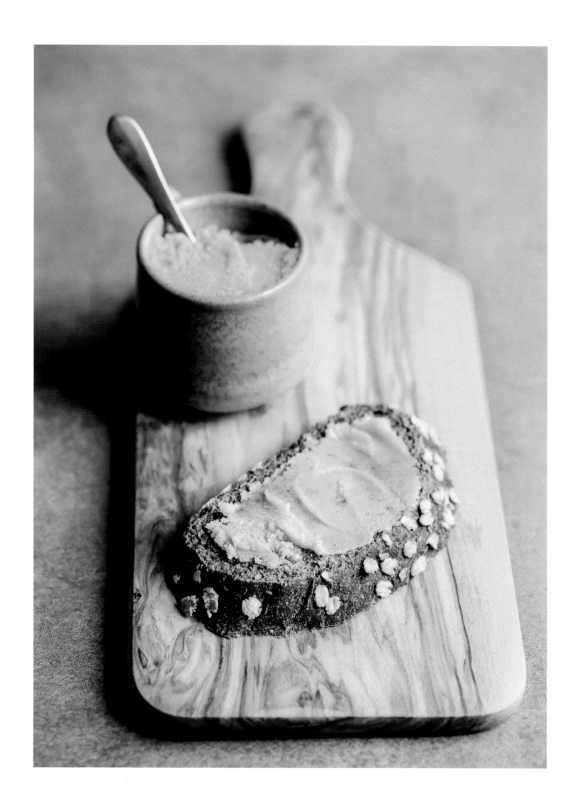

# ROSEMARY ROASTING GHEE

*MAKES 12 OUNCES*  Rosemary is slightly stimulating, which improves mental function and circulation. This is a great cooking oil for cool or cloudy weather to keep flavors bright. Making a garden-herb ghee will help you get ghee into your diet, especially if you are not used to Indian-style flavors. Try using this for roasting root vegetables (my favorite!) or for soups or even steamed vegetables. You can also go for *herbes de Provence* here.

**12 oz ghee**

**½ cup dried rosemary**

In a heavy-bottomed pan over medium-low heat, melt the ghee.

Add the rosemary, stir, and simmer until the mixture sizzles. Continue to sauté for 2 minutes, until fragrant. Remove from the heat and let cool.

Strain the ghee through a triple layer of cheesecloth to remove the herb into a clean, sterilized glass jar with a lid.

Keep the ghee at room temperature for up to 3 months, if it lasts that long!

### TIPS ON MAKING A DECOCTION

To make a decoction, start out with a wide saucepan so the water will evaporate more quickly. Be sure to use low heat so you do not burn the herb. The herb must be boiled in water until the water has reduced to one quarter of the original amount. This takes 1–2 hours. A fun trick for measuring this is to stand a wooden spoon in the pot with the water. Mark the handle where the water comes up to, and make another mark that denotes one quarter of the first mark. Use this measure to check as the water goes down, and remove from the heat when the water has been reduced to the one-quarter mark. You can use that spoon every time you make a decoction.

# BRAHMI GHEE

*MAKES 16 OUNCES*  Brahmi is a bitter, green herb, a relative of gotu kola, which is widely known as a support for memory and cognitive health. The root mass, a ball of finely twisting and interweaving threads, even reminds one of a brain. Because brahmi is so light in quality, mixing it with dense fats helps the herbal qualities nourish the brain. As a cooling rejuvenator for the mind, brahmi is also helpful for improving relaxation and sleep. This herb is the number-one choice to improve mental function, preserve a sharp intellect and quick recall, and protect the longevity of cognitive functions. I use it when I am working on a book! Due to its slightly bitter taste, taking a teaspoon of this ghee daily with a bit of milk will be most palatable.

¾ cup brahmi powder

2 qts water

16 oz ghee

**MAKE THE BRAHMI DECOCTION**

In a wide saucepan over medium-low heat, combine the brahmi and water and boil the mixture slowly, uncovered, until the water is reduced to one quarter (16 oz). Do not use high heat, as it can burn the herbs. This may take 1–2 hours. Strain the herb out using a double layer of cheesecloth inside a large metal strainer to hold the shape. Discard the herbs.

*Note:* See Tips on Making a Decoction on page 238.

**INFUSE THE GHEE**

In a large, wide pan over low heat, add the ghee and decoction and bring to a boil.

Simmer until all the water has evaporated. You will be able to see and hear (like popcorn) the water bubbles disappearing. When it is finished, there will be no water bubbles and no popping sounds. This may take 2 hours.

Allow the ghee to cool completely and transfer to a sterile glass jar with a tight lid.

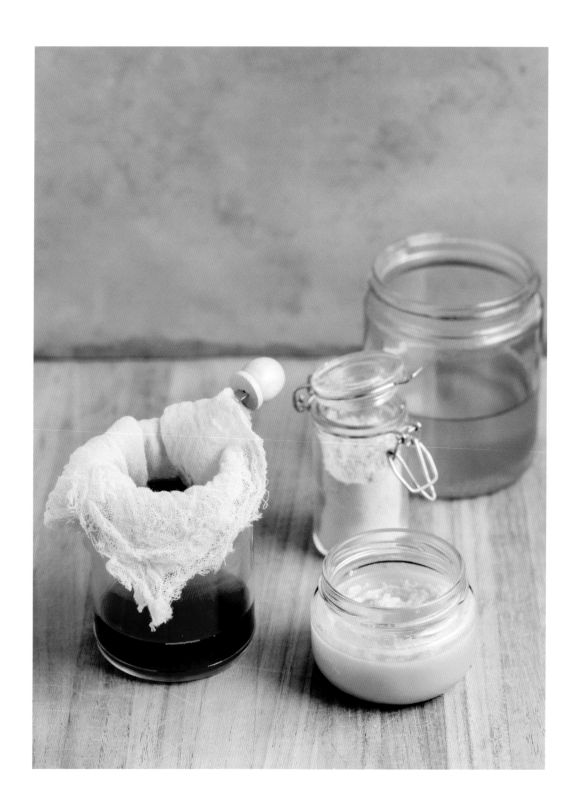

# SHATAVARI GHEE

*MAKES 16 OUNCES*  Shatavari ghee is most often used to support the female reproductive system, but men benefit as well. The herb is cooling and calming and has moist, heavy, dense qualities that protect and preserve the youth of the womb, eggs, sperm, breasts, and lactation. As a rejuvenating herb, shatavari supports pre- and postnatal health, and increases energy and immunity for everybody. Taking a teaspoon daily in a bit of hot milk or almond milk is best. A sprinkle of cinnamon or cardamom will make it more delicious, and it's not out of the question to have it on toast.

¾ cup shatavari powder

2 qts water

16 oz ghee

**MAKE THE SHATAVARI DECOCTION**

In a wide saucepan over medium-low heat, combine the shatavari and water, and boil the mixture slowly, uncovered, until the water is reduced to one quarter (16 oz). Do not use high heat, as it can burn the herbs. This may take 1–2 hours.

Strain the herb out using a double layer of cheesecloth inside a large metal strainer to hold the shape. Because shatavari is so unctuous, you may have to move the herbs around with a large spoon to keep it straining. The decoction will be thick. Discard the herbs.

**INFUSE THE GHEE**

In a large, wide pan over low heat, bring the ghee and decoction to a boil.

Simmer until all the water has evaporated. You will be able to see and hear (like popcorn) the water bubbles disappearing. When it is finished, there will be no water bubbles and no popping sounds. This may take 2 hours. Look closely for any water bubbles; if there is still water in your ghee, it will spoil.

Allow the ghee to cool completely and transfer to a sterile glass jar with a tight lid.

*Note:* Shatavari is a phytoestrogen, like soy, and is not recommended when there is a history of or genetic factor for breast cancer.

# ASHWAGANDHA GHEE

*MAKES 16 OUNCES* Ashwagandha ghee is an anti-aging nectar. Favored in winter for its warming virya, this rejuvenator supports the body during stress. *Ashva* means horse in Sanskrit, and this herb brings the strength of a horse. Infusing the herb into ghee targets reproductive health, especially for men, and brings virility and longevity to the organs. If you suffer in winter, travel a lot, or are just going through a difficult time, working a teaspoon of ashwagandha ghee into your diet daily will help you feel strong and protect the body from wear and tear.

¾ cup ashwagandha powder

2 qts water

16 oz ghee

### MAKE THE ASHWAGANDHA DECOCTION

In a wide saucepan over medium-low heat, combine the ashwagandha and water and boil the mixture slowly, uncovered, until the water is reduced to one quarter (16 oz). Do not use high heat, as it can burn the herbs. This may take 1–2 hours. Strain the herb out using a double layer of cheesecloth inside a large metal strainer to hold the shape. Discard the herbs.

### INFUSE THE GHEE

In a large, wide pan over low heat, add the ghee and decoction, and bring to a boil.

Simmer until all the water has evaporated. You will be able to see and hear (like popcorn) the water bubbles disappearing. When it is finished, there will be no water bubbles and no popping sounds. This may take 2 hours.

Allow the ghee to cool completely and transfer to a sterile glass jar with a tight lid.

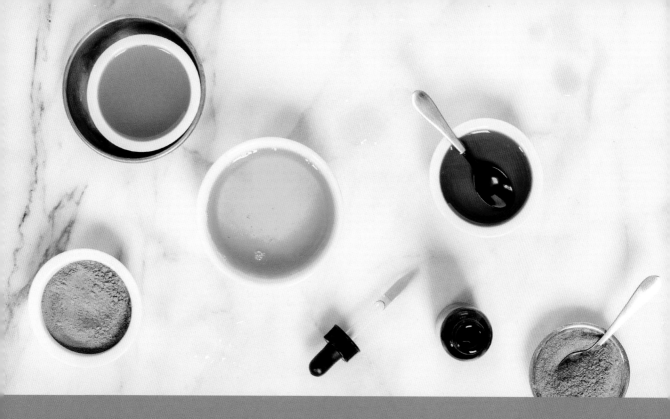

# THAILAM (HERBAL MASSAGE OILS)

A *thailam* is a base oil, such as sesame, coconut, or sunflower, that has been cooked along with an herbal decoction to make a "medicated oil." There is a wide variety of medicated oils for external, and sometimes internal, uses, and these oils are an important part of Ayurvedic treatment. One thailam can contain dozens of herbs. Using an herbal oil for self-massage can add targeted, concentrated benefits for the mind and the body. Herbs can increase oil's cooling or warming potency, change its density, and promote an herb's specific actions, such as calming the mind or soothing inflammation. All of these factors bring specific changes to your system.

**STARTING OUT.** Making herbal oils, like making herbal ghee, requires making a decoction first, to yield the herb's water-soluble qualities into a strong tea. The tea and the oil are then simmered together until all of the water has evaporated, which leaves the oil and the herb.

It's OK to start out with either refined or unrefined oils. Unrefined oils tend to be fresher. When you make an herbal oil, the cooking process will refine the oil again. Buy organic, small-batch oils from reputable suppliers. Store in colored glass or opaque plastic to keep light from aging the oils. Always keep your oils in a cool, dark place, out of the sun. These oils last for up to one year.

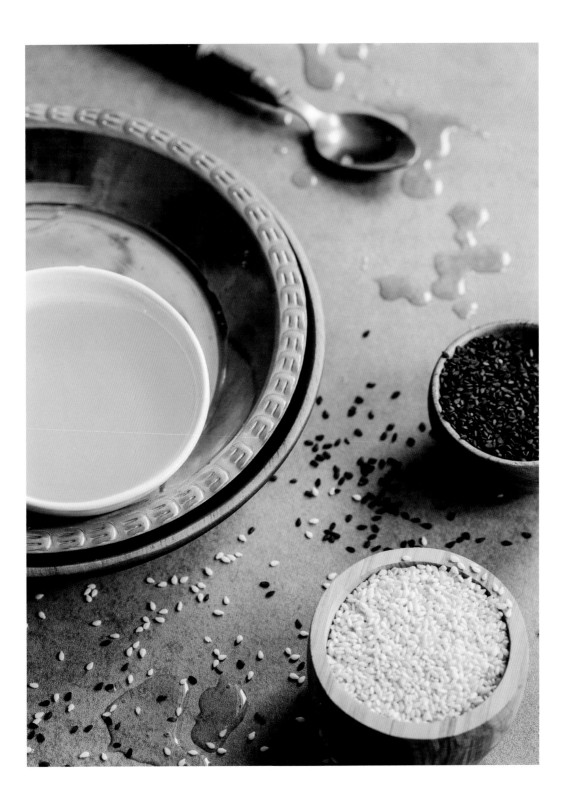

# BASIC CURED SESAME OIL

*MAKES 16 OUNCES*  Sesame oil is the richest and most age-fighting of the oils. The dry quality increases as we age, and sesame is the antidote. Not everyone tolerates sesame oil well, however, or needs its dense, warming properties. You will find massage oil for your body type in the box below. This sesame oil can be used for oiling ears, nose, feet, and mouth, as well as for body massage. You can also buy already-cured oil, which is called "refined." Curing at home makes it fresh, pure, and more easily absorbed by the skin. I find the texture of home-cured oils to be superior.

**16 oz unrefined sesame oil**

**Drop of water**

In a medium saucepan over medium-low heat, warm the oil just until it begins to move around in the pan.

Add a single drop of water into the oil; when it sizzles and disappears, the oil is done.

Remove from the heat and cool completely. Store the oil in a clean, dry vessel, preferably with a dispenser, such as an olive oil bottle.

## USING ESSENTIAL OILS

Essential oils are not traditionally used in thailam because scents are imparted to the oils from the herbal infusion. When using herbal oils, it's nice to smell the oil and the herbs alone. Essential oils, however, have their own concentrated qualities that can affect the body through sense of smell. They can be uplifting, grounding, or calming. If you are new to using natural oils on your skin, a little scent might help you get used to it. Here are a few suggestions.

**Grounding sesame oil**: If you run cold or have very dry skin, follow this recipe using sesame oil. Sesame oil is heavy and warming and best for cold weather. Use lavender, clary sage, or rosemary oil.

**Calming coconut oil**: If you run hot, have sensitive skin, or live in a very hot climate, use coconut oil mixed with sandalwood, rose, or lavender oil.

**Stimulating sunflower oil**: If you have a heavier constitution but still have dry skin, use sunflower oil. Add a citrus, eucalyptus, or lemongrass essential oil if you like. Sunflower oil can also be used by cold types who don't feel that sesame oil dissolves easily on the skin. Hot types can also use sunflower oil in cold and dry weather.

# TRIPHALA MASSAGE OIL

*MAKES 16 OUNCES*  Triphala does it all and is beneficial for all body types. Infusing massage oil with this triple-fruit compound increases its penetrating and rejuvenating qualities. The use of essential oils is optional and may inspire you to use your homemade product more often. Traditionally, herbal oils are scented by the herbs, not by additional oils. To get the scoop on choosing the right base oil for your body, see the section on abhyanga (page 82).

¾ cup triphala powder

2 qts water

16 oz coconut, sesame, or sunflower oil

10 drops essential oil (optional)

**MAKE THE TRIPHALA DECOCTION**

In a wide saucepan over medium-low heat, combine the triphala and water, and boil the mixture slowly, uncovered, until the water is reduced to one quarter (16 oz). Do not use high heat, as it can burn the herbs. This may take 1–2 hours. Strain the herb out using a triple layer of cheesecloth inside a large metal strainer to hold the shape. Discard the herbs.

**INFUSE THE OIL**

In a large, wide pan over low heat, add the oil and decoction, and bring to a boil.

Simmer until all the water has evaporated. You will be able to see and hear (like popcorn) the water bubbles disappearing. When it is finished, there will be no water bubbles and no popping sounds. Stir to be sure. This may take 2 hours.

Allow the oil to cool completely and transfer to a sterile glass jar with a tight lid.

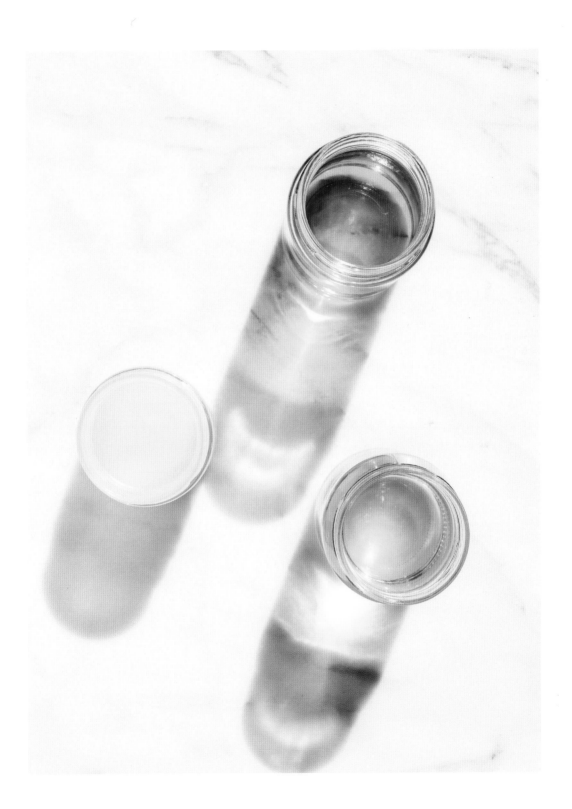

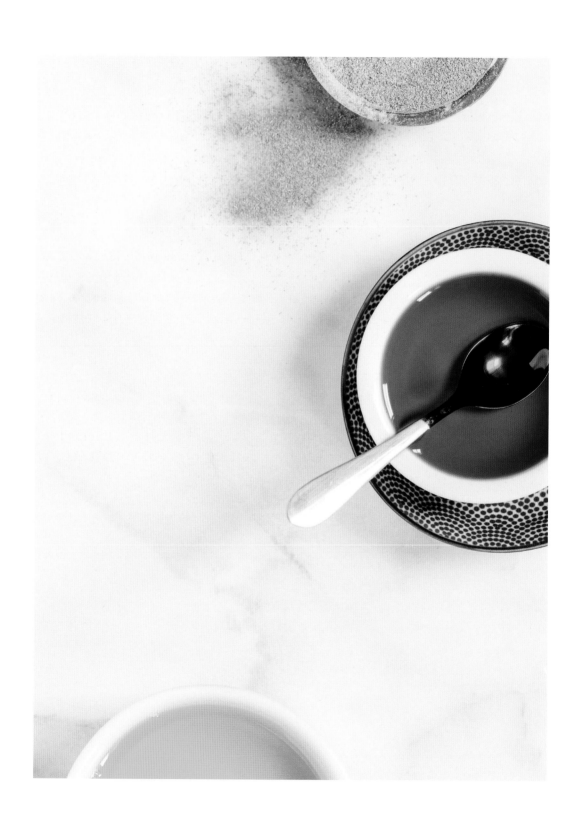

# STRESS-EASE BRAHMI OIL

*MAKES 16 OUNCES*  Brahmi's affinity for the brain and nervous system means it shows up in many medicines for the mind. A brahmi oil massage can cool and calm the body, nourish the nerves, and slow down an overactive mind. Use a sesame oil base if you run cold, have dry skin, or experience anxiety and fear due to stress. Use coconut oil if you run hot or get inflamed and irritated by stress. Be sure to include oiling of the head, ears, and nose.

¾ cup brahmi
powder

2 qts water

16 oz coconut or
sesame oil

### MAKE THE DECOCTION
In a wide saucepan over medium-low heat, combine the brahmi and water and boil the mixture slowly, uncovered, until the water is reduced to one quarter (16 oz). Do not use high heat, as it can burn the herbs. This may take 1–2 hours. Strain the herb out using a triple layer of cheesecloth inside a large metal strainer to hold the shape. Discard the herbs.

### INFUSE THE OIL
In a large, wide pan over low heat, add the oil and decoction, and bring to a boil.

Simmer until all the water has evaporated. You will be able to see and hear (like popcorn) the water bubbles disappearing. When it is finished, there will be no water bubbles and no popping sounds. Stir to be sure. This may take 2 hours.

Allow the oil to cool completely and transfer to a sterile glass jar with a tight lid.

# COOLING NEEM MASSAGE OIL

*MAKES 16 OUNCES* Neem is one of the more cooling herbs and is often used to cool down an overheated system. A neem oil massage will cool the blood, reduce inflammation and reactivity, relax and calm the mind, and reduce skin rashes and dry, itchy patches.

¾ cup neem powder

2 qts water

16 oz coconut oil

10 drops essential oil (optional)

**MAKE THE NEEM DECOCTION**

In a wide saucepan over medium-low heat, combine the herb and water and boil the mixture slowly, uncovered, until the water is reduced to one quarter (16 oz). Do not use high heat, as it can burn the herbs. This may take 1–2 hours. Strain the herb out using a triple layer of cheesecloth inside a large metal strainer to hold the shape. Discard the herbs.

**INFUSE THE OIL**

In a large, wide pan, add the oil and decoction, and bring to a boil.

Simmer until all the water has evaporated. You will be able to see and hear (like popcorn) the water bubbles disappearing. When it is finished, there will be no water bubbles and no popping sounds. Stir to be sure. This may take 2 hours.

Allow the oil to cool completely and transfer to a sterile glass jar with a tight lid. Favor a wide-mouth jar, as this oil will solidify in cooler temperatures.

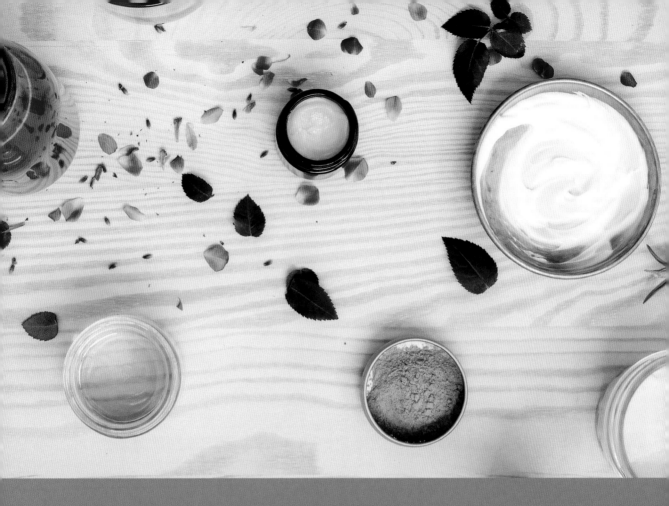

# BEAUTY TONICS AND TOPICALS

Did you know that more than half of what you put on your skin ends up in your bloodstream? Anything absorbed by your skin should be of a quality that would also be welcome in your mouth. This is pretty far from many of the products out there that can adversely affect not only our bodies but also our watersheds, as they ultimately get washed down the drain. I'm pretty passionate about using natural products in the bath. This section contains some of my favorite natural cleansing, toning, and nourishing tonics. It is such a pleasure to share them with you.

You probably see by now how Ayurveda considers external health a product of internal health. The skin, the largest of our sense organs, can show signs of stress and aging that are exposed to the eye in a way the internal skin (our digestive mucous membranes) is not. If you see dry quality or heat being expressed by the skin, it usually signals the same on the inside. Keep in mind that topical care of the skin is only part of the path to maintaining lustrous, clear, and youthful skin.

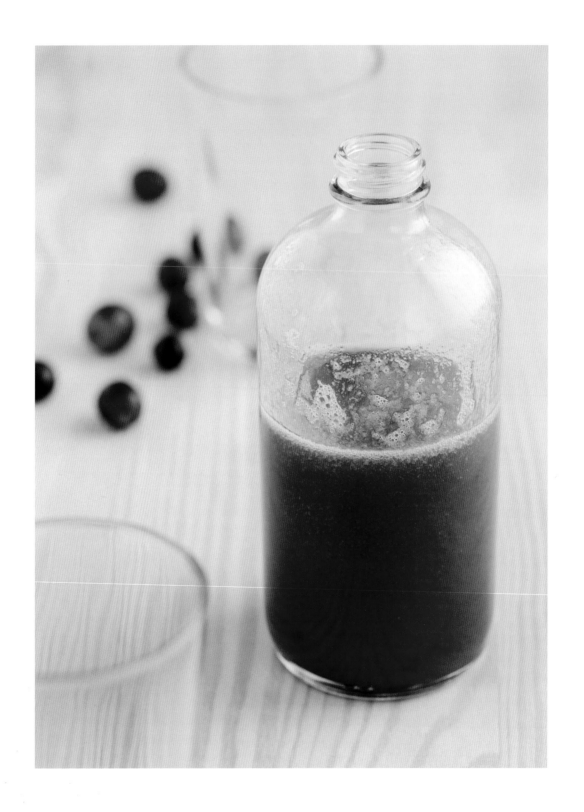

# CARDAMOM-GINGER GRAPE ELIXIR

*SERVES 2*  Many skin issues are actually a response to what's going on *beneath* the skin. This elixir both cleanses and nourishes the blood. Grapes are, in Ayurveda, "king among fruits." This fruit (the red ones, not the green ones) has the ability to nourish the rasa dhatu while cooling the rakta dhatu, which makes it an ideal rejuvenator for the blood. The addition of digestive spices brings a cleansing bonus for the upper digestive tract. Enjoy this juice often in hot weather, around the menstrual cycle, or to balance too much heating food yesterday. Try this instead of afternoon coffee (which will heat and dry the dhatus).

2 cups red
seedless grapes

½ cup water

¼ tsp ground
cardamom

1 tsp ground ginger

Lime wedges, for
garnish

Soak the grapes in cool water for 5 minutes, then drain and rinse.

Add the grapes, water, cardamom, and ginger to a blender, and blend on high for 1 minute, until smooth.

Strain through a metal sieve into tall glasses, using the back of a large spoon to press the juice through.

Alternatively, enjoy smoothie-style without straining.

Serve with a lime wedge.

---

### SMOOTHIE FOR SKIN

Check out Radiance Saffron-Almond Milk (page 209) for a nourishing tonic that brings luster to dry skin.

# THREE DIY FACIAL PACKS FOR YOUR SKIN TYPE

DIY facials are a luxurious yet simple weekly routine that brings luster and longevity to the skin. In addition, taking the time to care for your face brings that nourishing sensation of self-care that destresses and supports everyday living. I like to think of facial care as a two-birds-with-one-stone kind of thing that cultivates beauty inside and out. For optimal results, lie down and meditate on relaxing the eyes (especially the space between the eyebrows), the ears, the scalp, and the jaw while you let your mask sink in. It's a nice feeling!

Each of these recipes makes two applications, so get a friend! You can keep extra in the refrigerator for up to one week.

## SESAME PACK FOR DRY, UNDERNOURISHED SKIN

Sesame oil is the richest of the oils mentioned in traditional Ayurveda texts. Its slightly warming quality nourishes and penetrates very dry skin. Adding toning triphala powder and calming lavender makes this face pack a full-body experience that nourishes the mind as well as the skin. Tension shows in the face and, over time, can begin to age the skin. Relax the face for optimal absorption.

1 tbsp yogurt (at room temperature)

Few drops of sesame oil

¼ tsp triphala powder

2 drops lavender essential oil

In a small bowl, mix together the yogurt, sesame oil, triphala, and lavender oil until smooth.
  For best results, place a hot, moist towel over the face for a few minutes.
  Remove the towel and apply the mask to moist face using wide upward strokes.
  Leave the mask on for 10–20 minutes, relaxing the muscles of the face. Breathe in the lavender.
  Wipe off gently with a warm, damp cloth, using wide upward strokes.

*Vegan variation:* Use 1 tbsp ripe, mashed avocado instead of yogurt.

## TURMERIC AND NEEM PACK FOR BREAKOUTS OR COMBINATION SKIN

Chickpea flour exfoliates and dries pimples, while neem and turmeric cool and calm aggravated skin. If you don't have neem, make this mask with just turmeric. *(continued on page 256)*

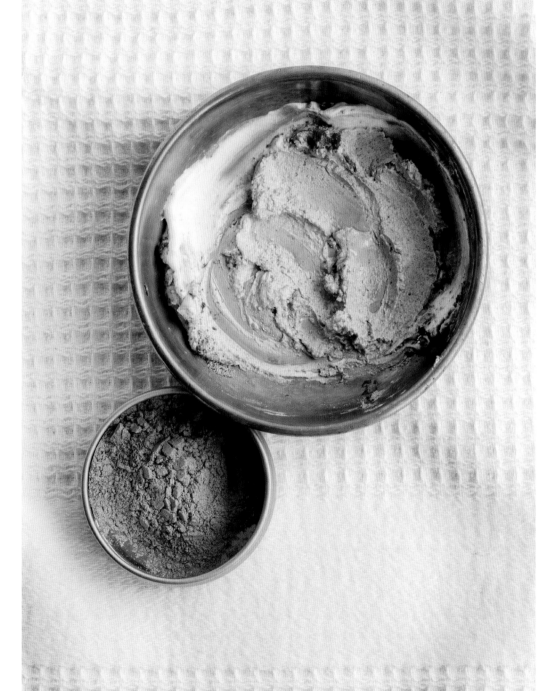

1 tbsp chickpea flour

¼ tsp neem powder

¼ tsp ground turmeric

1 tbsp water, aloe juice, or almond milk

In a small bowl, mix together the flour, neem, and turmeric.

Add the liquid and stir until a smooth paste forms.

Apply to the face using wide upward strokes.

Leave the mask on for 10–20 minutes, and enjoy the cooling sensation.

Wipe off gently with a damp cloth, using wide upward strokes.

---

## STIMULATING HONEY-BESAN PACK FOR DULL OR OILY SKIN

*Besan*, or chickpea flour, dries excess oil, while honey stimulates the skin and encourages blood flow. Triphala's astringent quality tones pores. Turmeric and saffron encourage a healthy glow.

1 tbsp yogurt

1 tsp honey

1 tbsp chickpea flour

¼ tsp triphala powder

¼ tsp ground turmeric or pinch of saffron threads

In a small bowl, mix together the yogurt and honey. Allowing the yogurt to warm to room temperature first will make this easier.

Add the chickpea flour, triphala, and turmeric, and stir until combined.

Apply to the face using wide upward strokes.

Leave the mask on for 10–20 minutes, and enjoy the cooling sensation.

Wipe off gently with a damp cloth, using wide upward strokes.

As a cleanser for oily skin, keep a mixture of six parts chickpea flour to one part ground turmeric at the ready. Place a spoonful in the palm and add a little hot water from the tap to make a paste. Massage the face gently with upward circling motions. Rinse clean. This one is great for teens who are going through an oily, acne-prone period.

# GHEE JOINT BALM

This recipe was contributed by the Boston-based Ayurvedic practitioner Veronica Wolff-Casey. The easy-to-make mixture of ghee and turmeric calms and reduces inflammation in overworked joints. Try this for ankles, wrists, and knees, and be sure to cover the treated area with plastic wrap to avoid staining anything.

**2 tsp ground turmeric**

**1 tbsp ghee**

In a small bowl, combine the turmeric and ghee until the consistency becomes like smooth peanut butter.

Apply the oily paste to the joint, and rub it deeply into the area.

Wrap with plastic wrap and keep it on overnight. Wash the balm off in the morning. The turmeric will leave a yellow color on the skin for a few hours.

Repeat for a few nights or until pain diminishes.

This balm will keep for 3 months on the shelf and 1 year in the refrigerator.

## NEEM FACIAL BALM

Try using Cooling Neem Massage Oil (page 250) as a facial balm in humid hot weather or for acne-prone skin and irritated or itchy patches.

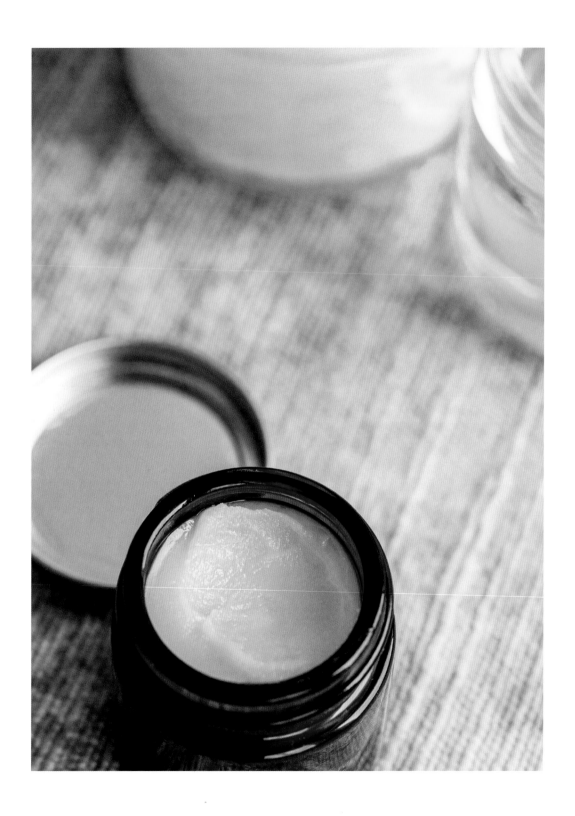

# GHEE FACIAL BALM

The creator of Birchstone Apothecary was a student in my Ayurveda school, and she gifted me a sample of an herbal facial balm she created using ghee as the base. I stuck it in my travel bag, and now I'm hooked. Amy was kind enough to develop a similar recipe for you all to make at home. Ghee offers deep moisture for dry skin, as well as cooling qualities for inflamed and sensitive areas. This balm can be used as an eye cream or night cream, as well as a salve for dry patches, healing scabs, ragged cuticles, and calloused feet.

2 oz ghee

2 oz refined organic sesame oil

½ oz beeswax

16–30 drops rose or sandalwood essential oil (optional)

Add the ghee, sesame oil, and beeswax to a 16-oz wide-mouth jar.

Fill a small pot with 1–2 inches of water and place over medium heat.

Set the jar full of ingredients in the water until the contents are thoroughly melted, about 15 minutes, swirling occasionally.

If adding essential oils, allow the mixture to cool for several minutes first, until the jar is warm (but not hot) to the touch. Add in your favorite essential oil or essential oil blend and mix thoroughly with a spoon.

Pour the mixture into a sterilized 4-oz glass jar and let it stand with the lid off until completely cool and nearly solid. In hot weather, it will remain a little soft.

Scoop out a small amount of balm with clean fingertips and massage it into the skin until thoroughly absorbed. Use from head to toe to hydrate and nourish dry skin. A little bit will go a long way!

Store in a cool, dry place and use within 6–8 months.

# CASTOR OIL PACK

The external use of castor oil is ancient and worldwide. The oil's qualities are incredibly heavy, moist, and penetrating. This recipe's combination allows castor oil to break up physical and energetic blockages and move stagnation (that's why it's a strong laxative!). Packs are helpful for inflamed joints, constipation, back pain, and painful periods. You can find castor oil for external use in a natural foods store with the body oils or online from one of the suppliers in the Resources section. Hot water bottles can be purchased at any pharmacy.

3 tbsp castor oil

Hot water bottle

Piece of flannel, at least 18 square inches, or a cut-up old T-shirt or pillowcase

Plastic bag or plastic wrap (a shopping bag will do)

Warm the castor oil by standing the bottle in a pan or sink of hot water for 5 minutes.

Fill the hot water bottle two-thirds full with very hot water. Press a bit of the air out before screwing on the cap tightly. This will make the bottle less hard so it stays put.

Fold the cloth into a rectangle that will cover the affected area. For constipation or painful periods, the area is between the hip bones, from the navel to the pubic bone. For back pain, cover an area at least 6–8 square inches, not just the localized place of pain.

Dampen one side of the cloth with castor oil. It should be very moist but not dripping.

Place the cloth over the area and cover it with a plastic bag or piece of plastic wrap.

Place the hot water bottle over the plastic and the cloth.

Rest with the pack on for 60–90 minutes. A longer application will get faster results. Take a hot shower and wash the area twice with soap to remove the oil. Swabbing with a solution of baking soda and water will also remove it. Castor oil does stain, so take care.

## OIL THE KNEES

My yoga teacher always recommended castor oil for pain in the knees. It works. It also breaks up scar tissue, so postinjury, castor oil applications can help you maintain mobility in the long term. Warm oil can be applied directly to the skin and massaged in well. Wrap the knee(s) with plastic wrap to protect bedsheets and clothing. Rest with hot water bottles or a heating pad over the knees. Keep this on for 1 hour, or apply at night and sleep with it on. Wash in the morning with hot water and soap to remove the oil. Do this daily until the pain is gone.

The pack can be stored in a sealed sandwich bag in the freezer between uses.

*Notes:* For painful periods, do this daily, but *not* when you are having your period. Within a month or two, you should notice a difference. For constipation, do this daily until things are moving. Resort back as needed for chronic constipation.

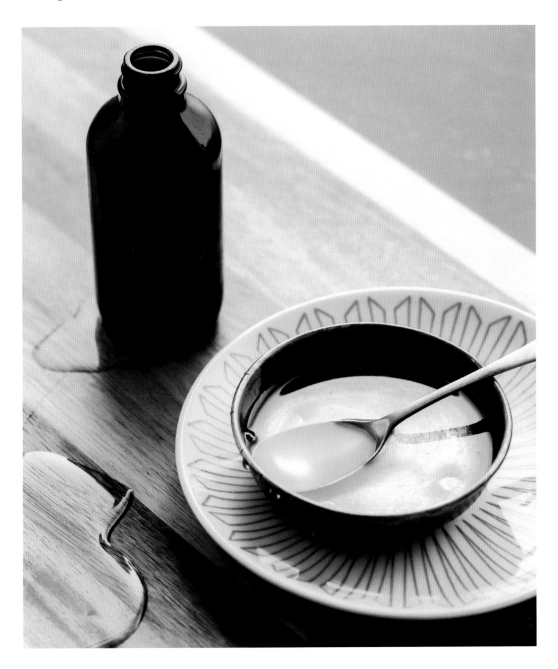

# GLOSSARY

## SANSKRIT TERMS

**Abyhanga:** Warm oil massage.

**Agni:** The fire element; the principle of transformation in the body.

**Ahara rasa:** Literally "juice of the food"; the nutritive liquid resulting from food being broken down in the stomach.

**Ama:** Toxicity in the body resulting from undigested food, experience, and emotion.

**Anupana:** Material, usually a liquid, that is consumed along with a medicine to enhance the efficacy of that medicine.

**Ashtanga Hrdayam:** An abridged compilation of the Charaka Samhita written by Vagbhata.

**Atman:** Soul.

**Buddhi:** Intellect; a faculty of the mind.

**Charaka Samhita:** The most commonly used foundational text on Ayurveda in Sanskrit, likely written by a compilation of people at least two thousand years ago.

**Citta:** Field of awareness; includes the subconscious.

**Deepana:** The action of kindling digestive fire.

**Dhatu:** That which maintains as well as nourishes the body; the seven tissue types.

**Dinacharya:** The daily cycles of nature; daily routine.

**Dosha:** Literally "that which is at fault"; essential biological compounds present in the body.

**Guna:** Strand; quality.

**Indriyas:** The senses.

**Jathara agni:** The digestive fire in the stomach; mother of all agnis.

**Jnanendriyas:** Organs of knowledge.

**Kala:** Time, specifically time of day, time of year, and time of life.

**Kanjee:** A thin gruel made from rice and water.

**Kapha:** The energy of cohesion.

**Karma:** Action.

**Karmendriyas:** Organs of action.

**Kashayam:** An herbal preparation made by boiling herbs over low heat for several hours.

**Mala:** Impurity; a waste product.

**Manas:** Mind.

**Maya:** The illusion or appearance of the manifest world.

**Nasya:** The administration of medicines through the nasal cavity.

**Ojas:** Literally "vigor"; the cream of the nutrient fluid in the body; the final product of digestion; the essence of immunity.

**Pachana:** The action of improving digestion and absorption.

**Parinama:** Change.

**Pitta:** That which transforms or digests.

**Prabhava:** A special action of a substance that is not easily explained by its qualities.

**Prajnaparadha:** A crime against intelligence; a malfunction of the mental faculties.

**Prakriti:** Literally "nature"; personal constitution; individual makeup of the five elements and three doshas.

**Prana:** The vital energy of the universe.

**Purusha:** Cosmic consciousness; universal principle.

**Rasa:** Literally "sap," "juice," or "mood"; refers to the classification of taste according to the qualities of a substance, as in shad rasa.

**Rasayana:** Literally "path of essence"; science of longevity; a group of herbal medicines used to promote longevity.

**Ritucharya:** Seasonal routine.

**Samprapti:** Knowledge of the pathways of disease manifestation.

**Sankhya:** One of the six major schools of Indian philosophy; presents a systematic ontology of the cosmos having twenty-five categories.

**Sattva:** A clear and undisturbed state of mind; synonym for "mind."

**Shad rasa:** Six tastes—sweet, sour, salty, pungent, bitter, and astringent—used to classify foods and medicines according to qualities.

**Shamana:** Pacification of the doshas.

**Shiro-abhyanga:** Head massage with oil.

**Shodhana:** Cleansing or purification; a forcible removal of dosha.

**Srotamsi:** Plural of srotas.

**Srotas:** Channel; transportation system of the body.

**Swastha:** To be seated in the self; a synonym for "health."

**Takra:** Ayurvedic buttermilk, made by churning yogurt in water.

**Tanmatras:** The subtle elements that are the objects of the five senses.

**Tridoshic:** Quality of a substance that does not cause imbalance in any of the three doshas.

**Trividha karana:** Three main causes of disease.

**Vata:** That which moves.

**Vipaka:** Postdigestive effect; the effect a substance has on the digestive tract after being processed in the stomach.

**Virya:** The ultimate potency of a substance; the effect on the body of heating or cooling.

# NOTES

---

## INTRODUCTION
1. Charaka Samhita, Sutrasthana, 1.42.

## CHAPTER 1. WHAT YOU NEED TO KNOW ABOUT AYURVEDA
1. Vagbhata, Ashtanga Hrdayam, Sutrasthana, 1.6: "The dosha are material substances in the body always, they have their own definite quantity, quality, and functions. When they are normal they attend to different functions of the body and so maintain it. But they have the tendency to become abnormal undergoing increase or decrease in their quantity, one or more of their qualities and functions… because of this tendency to vitiation (disorder), they are called as doshas."
2. Vagbhata, Ashtanga Hrdayam, Sutrasthana, 12.40–42.

## CHAPTER 2. THE PHYSICAL BODY
1. Charaka Samhita, Sarirasthana, vol. 2, 7.15.
2. Charaka Samhita, Sarirasthana, vol. 2, 3.12.
3. Charaka Samhita, Vimanasthana, 5.7–8.
4. Charaka Samhita, Vimanasthana, 5.7–8.
5. Claudia Welch, *Secrets of the Mind* (Darling Point, Australia: Big Shakti, 2005). https://drclaudiawelch.com/wp-content/uploads/2016/07/Secrets_of_the_Mind_ebook.pdf.
6. Charaka Samhita, Sutrasthana, 30.1–15.

## CHAPTER 3. THE MIND
1. Charaka Samhita, Sutrasthana, vol. 1, 30.13–14.

## CHAPTER 4. THE SUBTLE BODY
1. Charaka Samhita, Sutrasthana, 30.9.

## CHAPTER 5. DINACHARYA
1. Charaka Samhita, Sutrasthana, 5.85–89.
2. Vagbhata, Ashtanga Hrdayam, Sutrasthana, 2.10–11.

## CHAPTER 6. RITUCHARYA
1. Vagbhata, Ashtanga Hrdayam, Uttarasthana, 39.4.

## CHAPTER 10. HOME REMEDIES
1. Vagbhata, Ashtanga Hrdayam, Sutrasthana, 5.18.
2. Talya's Feel Better Tea recipe was printed by permission of Talya Lutzker. Copyright © Talya Lutzker and Talya's Kitchen, 2018.
3. Vagbhata, Ashtanga Hrdayam, Sutrasthana, 5.37–39.

# RESOURCES

---

## SUPPLIERS OF AYURVEDIC GOODS

**The Ayurvedic Institute**
Herbs, herbal ghees, massage oils, nasya oil
www.ayurveda.com/products

**Banyan Botanicals**
Herbs and spices, massage oils, dinacharya supplies
www.banyanbotanicals.com

**Birchstone Apothecary**
Small-batch skincare products handmade in New England
www.birchstoneapothecary.com

**Mountain Rose Herbs**
Herbs, spices, and essential oils
www.mountainroseherbs.com

**Pukka Herbs**
Ayurvedic teas, herbal products
www.pukkaherbs.us (US); www.pukkaherbs.com (UK)

**Pure Indian Foods**
Herbal ghees, cultured ghee, Ayurvedic herbs, spices, oils, and sundries
www.pureindianfoods.com

**Rasasara Skinfood Australia**
Ayurvedic, small batch, herbal facial and hair care
https://rasasara.com

**Sarada Ayurvedic Remedies**
Handmade body and beauty products, massage oils, nasya oil
https://saradausa.com

## PRACTITIONER SOURCES

**National Ayurvedic Medical Association**
Directory of Ayurvedic practitioners
www.ayurvedanama.org (US); www.ayurveda-association.eu (Europe)

**Vaidyagrama Healing Village**
Panchakarma center in India
www.vaidyagrama.com

## READING LIST

Agnivesa. *Charaka Samhita*. Trans. Dr. Ram Karan Sharma and Vaidya Bhagwan Dash. Varanasi: Chowkhamba Krishnadas Academy, 2009.

Frawley, David. *The Yoga of Herbs*. Twin Lakes, WI: Lotus Press, 1986.

Lad, Vasant. *The Complete Book of Ayurvedic Home Remedies*. Albuquerque, NM: Ayurvedic Press, 1999.

——. *Textbook of Ayurveda: Fundamental Principles*. Albuquerque, NM: Ayurvedic Press, 2002.

Morningstar, Amadea. *Ayurvedic Cooking for Westerners*. Twin Lakes, WI: Lotus Press, 1995.

——. *Easy Healing Drinks*. Santa Fe, NM: Ayurveda Polarity Therapy & Yoga Institute with Nataraj Book, 2018. (eBook available at www.easyhealingdrinks.com.)

O'Donnell, Kate. *The Everyday Ayurveda Cookbook*. Boston: Shambhala Publications, 2014.

——. *Everyday Ayurveda Cooking for a Calm, Clear Mind*. Boulder, CO: Shambhala Publications, 2017.

Pole, Sebastian. *Ayurvedic Medicine: The Principles of Traditional Practice*. Philadelphia, PA: Singing Dragon, 2012.

Pursell, J. J. *The Herbal Apothecary*. Portland, OR: Timber Press, 2015.

Stillman, Cate. *Body Thrive*. Boulder, CO: Sounds True, 2018.

——. *Master of You: A Five-Point System to Synchronize Your Body, Your Home, and Your Time with Your Ambition*. Boulder, CO: Sounds True, 2020.

Svoboda, Robert E. *Prakriti*. Twin Lakes, WI: Lotus Press, 1998.

Vagbhata. *Ashtanga Hrdayam*. 6th ed. Trans. K. R. Srikantha Murthy. Varanasi, India: Chowkhamba Krishnadas Academy, 2009.

Welch, Claudia. *Balance Your Hormones, Balance Your Life*. Boston: Da Capo Lifelong Books, 2011.

# ACKNOWLEDGMENTS

I would like to thank the following people who were instrumental in the process of creating this book.

All the folks at Shambhala Publications for the vision and its execution.

Cara Brostrom, whose commitment to Ayurvedic living shows in her photography. Cara would also like to thank Kimberly Zane for ceramics used in the photos; Tara Sweeney, for acting as cooking assistant; and Adriana Christianson, for providing Indian wares for styling.

Carabeth Connelly, head recipe tester (and sometimes caterer), and the recipe testing team.

Great teachers Anusha Seghal, Sharathji Jois, Robert Svoboda, Scott Blossom, and Claudia Welch; the doctors at Vaidyagrama and its founder, Dr. Ramkumar.

My partner, Rich Ray, master of compassionate self-observation.

My bestie, Erin Casperson, for the Ayurvedic expert review—and for always being there in times of crisis.

The recipe contributors: Amadea Morningstar, Claudia Welch, Talya Lutzker, Erin Casperson, Cate Stillman, Cara Brostrom, and Veronica Wolff-Casey.

Those who support my work from behind the scenes, in ways that are obvious or not so obvious: Down Under Yoga, Boston Ayurveda School, the Kripalu Center, Linda Borman, Jim Rubenstein, Louise Giordanni, Didi Von Deck, Katie Bickford, Karen Kirkness, Uni Leroy Bunbun and Fudgey, my Ashtanga yoga students in both cities, and all those who attend my workshops in person and online.

All my readers, wherever you are—you bring my work to life.

# INDEX

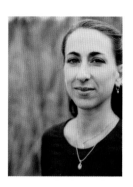

## ABOUT THE AUTHOR

**KATE O'DONNELL** is the author of three books published in five languages, as well as an international presenter, Ayurvedic practitioner, and senior Ashtanga yoga teacher. She is the founder of the Ayurvedic Living Institute, an online hub for education and resources for the Ayurvedic lifestyle. She lives in Portland, Maine, and can be reached at www.kateodonnell.yoga.

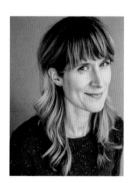

## ABOUT THE PHOTOGRAPHER

**CARA BROSTROM** is a lifestyle, editorial, and fine art photographer. As a visual storyteller, her photography documents the landscapes, objects, and moments that reveal our modern lives. She lives in Massachusetts with her family.
www.carabrostrom.com // @carabros

Shambhala Publications, Inc.
4720 Walnut Street
Boulder, Colorado 80301
www.shambhala.com

© 2020 by Kathleen O'Donnell
Photographs © 2020 by Cara Brostrom

Talya's Feel Better Tea recipe was printed by permission of Talya Lutzker, © 2018
by Talya Lutzker and Talya's Kitchen.

Cover photographs: Cara Brostrom
Cover design: Kate E. White
Interior design: Allison Meierding

9 8 7 6 5 4 3 2 1

First Edition
Printed in the United States of America

⊗ This edition is printed on acid-free paper that meets the
American National Standards Institute Z39.48 Standard.
♻ Shambhala Publications makes every effort to print on recycled paper.
For more information please visit www.shambhala.com.
Shambhala Publications is distributed worldwide by Penguin Random House, Inc.,
and its subsidiaries.

Library of Congress Cataloging-in-Publication Data
Names: O'Donnell, Kate (Ayurvedic practitioner) author.
Title: The everyday Ayurveda guide to self-care: rhythms, routines, and
home remedies for natural healing / Kate O'Donnell; photographs by Cara Brostrom.
Description: Boulder, Colorado: Shambhala, [2020] | Includes index.
Identifiers: LCCN 2019032537 | ISBN 9781611806519 (paperback)
Subjects: LCSH: Medicine, Ayurvedic. | Mind and body. | Self-care, Health. | Healing.
Classification: LCC R605 .O323 2020 | DDC 615.5/38—dc23
LC record available at https://lccn.loc.gov/2019032537

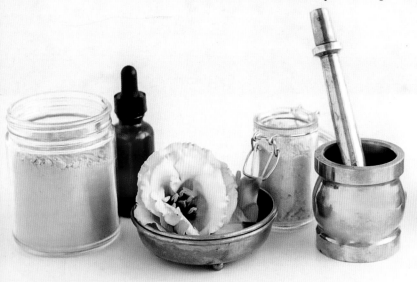
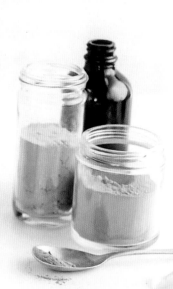